Autoimmune Survival Guide

ISBN: 978-1-77995-011-6
e-ISBN: 978-1-77995-012-3

First edition, first impression 2023

Published by Bookstorm (Pty) Ltd
PO Box 296
Riebeek Kasteel
Western Cape
7307
South Africa
www.bookstorm.co.za

Edited by Angela Voges
Proofread by Janet Bartlet
Cover design by Dogstar Design
Book design and typesetting by Dogstar Design
Printed by the USA

Autoimmune Survival Guide

Support for people suffering from
autoimmune and other
trauma-driven conditions

Malvina Bartmanski

Dedication

This book is dedicated to my parents,
Margaret and Daniel, for creating the path and supporting me
while I both glide and tumble down it.
I also dedicate it to all the healer practitioners I have met
on my journey – all of my encounters shaped the pages of this book.
Some of these healers have even become valued friends. Some have been
other-worldly peak experiences and imprinted memorable words
in my mind such as:
"All sickness is soul sickness."
The healing journey has been my greatest adventure. Thank you.

Preface

I AM A CLINICAL PSYCHOLOGIST practising in South Africa, working dominantly with complex trauma and autoimmune conditions. Having found myself repeatedly explaining the contents of these pages to patients, I decided that perhaps there is a gap here that needs to be filled with a book.

I am finding that an ever-increasing number of people in my practice have been diagnosed with autoimmune and other stress- and trauma-related conditions. I have especially witnessed an increase in my practice of women needing integrative support for psychological and health concerns simultaneously in recent years. Many exhibit the beginnings of autoimmune symptoms without knowing it. As I am writing this, I can say that about 80 per cent of my current patients are experiencing autoimmune symptoms or already have a diagnosis. People don't know where to turn with these symptoms and the psychological impact they have. I have had my own health journey here; perhaps this was preparation for guiding many through theirs.

These conditions appear to have a strong psychological component in that they are linked to the experience of psychological trauma and stress. People often land up in my practice to address the trauma that seems to be at the origin of their health condition, usually unaware that this forms a big part of that condition. This is where the psychologist's role overlaps with that of the medical profession in the treatment of these conditions. Doctors often understand autoimmune disorders as something deficient with the immune system or driven by a pathogen such as a virus, fungus or bacterium (or often a combination of these), which is certainly true. However, I would like to introduce the idea that is coming up in much of the research in this area: that these disorders are driven by a nervous system dysregulated by trauma and stress. A traumatised nervous system then acts to suppress the healthy immune system, stopping it from doing what it would usually do quite well without any support and allowing pathogens to flourish.

This book aims to help you climb out of the autoimmunity black hole holistically and naturally, and perhaps even to fully restore your health. I had to figure out this healing path alone, but maybe this book can save you the trouble. I have written about the things that have helped me specifically, so this book certainly does not include every path of healing there is. It is for those affected by autoimmune conditions and symptoms, psychologists and other practitioners working in this space, as well as those interested in the link between body and mind.

 Task

I suggest that, while reading this book, you keep a notebook handy: there are some opportunities to do some investigative work into how this all began, and how to make your way out of it. Perhaps the first thing in this notebook can be a list of all your symptoms. My symptoms included brain fog, inability to concentrate, pelvic pain, mood swings, lower back pain, joint pain, nerve pain, headaches, breast cysts and a lump on my thyroid. Track these symptoms for changes once a month over the next few months while you implement some of the strategies in this book. This can help you check in and see whether the changes you are making are working, or whether you may need to refine them.

Contents

PART 1

Introduction to autoimmune and trauma-driven conditions

THIS BOOK AIMS to address the real pandemic that is presenting in society – a surge of autoimmune disease, burnout and hormonal dysregulation. More and more women in my practice are arriving with autoimmune manifestations or endocrine imbalances. I say women as this seems to affect far more women than men, from what I am seeing (or perhaps women are more help-seeking than men). It is rare these days for a person to arrive at my practice without some form of health difficulty.

What is driving this? I believe it is multiple things. Firstly, women's bodies are not designed to sustain survival mode for as long as men's bodies can (I will explain survival mode a bit later). From an evolutionary perspective, women were gatherers, men were hunters. Men would go out into the fields and chase animals, often not returning for some days and finding ways to survive out there in the wild. Men developed rational, strategic thinking and wisdom in this space. Women stayed in community with other women and children and focused on growing and gathering plants for food supply, nurturing and healing. Women developed intuition and emotional connection abilities in this space. They evolved to preserve relationships and connection, often at all costs.

Traditionally, men fulfilled the protector and provider role (or container) to their families and even the wider community. On returning from the wild they would receive care, healing, nurture and validation from the women in the community. This validation is what men often feel is missing in their lives in modern times – something I see regularly in my practice. Women feel neglected and disconnected, yearning for quality time with others; men feel criticised, and that their self-esteem is damaged – a loop that is unfortunately feeding itself, and that indicates an imbalance in our social systems.

If we look at life in society now, many women are living a life outside of their evolutionary path – running businesses, travelling the world for work, often with a family and household in the background too. Are their bodies able to cope with what they're trying do with them? I suspect men's bodies are better able to sustain high adrenaline and that their hormone systems aren't as sensitive as those of women due to their evolution. I don't want to upset any feminists here, so it is worth saying that I am certainly proud of women. About 100 years ago we had no rights, no work, no vote, nothing, without being owned by others. In my practice, women often mention that they don't have the quality time they would like to have with their partners and children. It is almost as though they are disconnected from their feminine nature. Gabor Maté mentions in this book, *The Myth of Normal*, that society reinforces men's sense of being entitled to women's care. Some men are aware of the care they receive only in its absence and experience intense resentment when it is withdrawn. He describes some of women's health symptoms as coming from absorption of male angst and the culturally directed responsibility for soothing it. Perhaps these increasing diagnoses in women are our bodies screaming out against these multiple roles embedded in a patriarchal society.

I believe that the imbalances between the feminine and the masculine are one of the things fuelling these accelerating diagnoses of autoimmunity. Another aspect of this is that many women seem to live in a perpetual state of fear. As the smaller of the sexes, we are generally more vulnerable than men. Many women in my practice mention feeling chronically unsafe; very few men ever mention this. There is truth in this: women's safety is frequently violated, especially in a country like South Africa where the statistics about this are astounding. Women are more regularly subject to sexual violations and trauma than men. Also in *The Myth of Normal*, Gabor Maté states that sexual harassment is a constant menace that women face. This is something we need to consider – that we have designed the world as a threatening place for women.

Something is driving autoimmunity at its source. Previous generations don't seem to have been as afflicted as recent ones. Autoimmunity doesn't discriminate age-wise any more either, in that twenty-something-year-olds who have barely begun their lives are frequently receiving these diagnoses. I have a sense that this is partly as a consequence of the microbiomes in the soil. A community of microorganisms, including eukaryotes, archaea, fungi, viruses and bacteria, that interact with and within a particular environment is known as a microbiome. It is, in essence, the balance of good and bad bacteria and pathogens. We have dysregulated the earth's microbiome, resulting in various pathogens (viruses, bacteria and fungi) mutating and becoming ever stronger. We could almost look at the world as a mirror of what is going on in most of our guts. There is an imbalance of good and bad 'bacteria', with the bad bacteria (and other pathogens) dominating. Our waters, our soils, our seas – everything is polluted or over-extended (or becoming so), out of its natural harmony. This disruption of the microbiome not only causes an increase in pathogens, but also decreases the level of nutrition available to us from the food growing in these damaged environments. We have disturbed the perfect balance of nature by not being conscious that each part of nature plays an important interconnected role in sustaining the functioning of the whole system, with us and our health forming part of this complex system.

Think about the kinds of soils our farmers are farming in. They are often over-farmed; where do plants get their nutrients from, if not the soil, the air and even the rain? What is the condition of this soil, air and rain? The soil microbiome governs the biogeochemical cycling of macronutrients, micronutrients and other elements vital for the growth of plants and animal life. We need to understand and predict the impact of climate change on soil microbiomes and the ecosystem, and begin to appreciate how interconnected we all are. Microbiomes are directly responsible for the health of the environment and the way it functions, collaborating to confer benefits that can help an organism thwart stressors and invaders, and making it more resilient overall. Conversely, when their composition is altered, their environment is altered, and the organisms in it can suffer as a result.

Research is beginning to indicate that our internal microbiome disruptions are mirroring what is taking place in the natural world. When the soil microbiome is balanced and healthy, it has a direct, positive impact on the health of the plants that grow there and shields them from pests and drought. When pathogens try to attack plants, a balanced microbiome may drive them away, produce toxins to kill them off and trigger the plants to defend themselves. The same molecules that are used for the health of a plant in soil are needed to maintain the balance in our gut. Soil and the human gut contain approximately the same number of active microorganisms, while human gut microbiome diversity is only 10 per cent of that of soil biodiversity and has decreased dramatically with the modern lifestyle. No man is an island – everything in nature exists in an interconnected, ancient, intelligent design. Gut microbes produce enzymes that help us digest food and break it down into essential nutrients, producing vitamins our own bodies cannot make on their own; protect us from disease-causing bacteria by regulating our immune system and teaching it how to fight off invaders; and produce anti-inflammatory compounds. Our microbiomes are unique, passed on from our mothers when we're born. Likewise, microbiomes in soil differ in composition depending on the region, type of soil, plant matter and a variety of other factors.

Despite all the powerful benefits they can confer, microbiomes are hardly invincible, and human activity has done much to disrupt them. The devastation of the soil microbiome is mostly a result of industrial farming practices. The soil and its plants suffer as these microorganisms disappear – and as we consume progressively fewer different kinds of microorganisms into our gut microbiomes, so does our health. Some of these microbes might genuinely be in danger of becoming extinct, which would have unknowable repercussions on human health. Our diets have become reliant on monocultures of processed and fatty foods that do not properly 'feed' our tenant microbes and keep them in balance, leaving us susceptible to diseases such as obesity, cancer and autoimmune conditions. As we've moved from being hunter-gatherers to living in an urbanised society, the human gut has lost its diversity. On top of our limited contact with soil and faeces, through our hygiene measures, the antibiotics we take and the low-fibre diets of processed foods we eat, we have lost beneficial microbes. These developments concur with an increase in autoimmune diseases that are related to the human intestinal microbiome.

The stress of living in our adrenaline-based society requires good nutrition. We are nutrient deficient, stressed and traumatised, living in environments full of pollutants in which pathogens like viruses can thrive. While the solution to this problem lies in repairing society and how we live, this book is focused on you as an individual and on getting to the unique root of what drives these conditions for you. But maybe it can also be activating enough to drive some collective change; our health and survival seem to be dependent on it.

Where do you start?

For those who are beginning to read this book in the midst of or discovering that there is something unwanted going on in their bodies, I salute you. I know you are scared. I have been there, and faced solving the complex health puzzle that this journey takes you on. The anxiety, the depression, and sometimes the bouts of denial that provide relief in this process that is peeling away all of your layers until you get to the core of what this is, who you are, who in life is behind you, and what you are made of. It may feel as if all your life plans have been shattered and the grief of that is weighing deeply on you.

Right now, put that all on the shelf. Let those plans wait. You are now on a detour, and I promise that when you look at those plans again one day they will have transformed. This is a time of internal focus. Life has sent you on a journey that will change everything you are and everything inside you – if you allow it to. You're on a very narrow pathway that isn't clearly lit yet, and you can't see the exit sign – but I promise it exists. Only you can find it, however. You will have to make this journey alone, following what you know to be best for you. It is a difficult experience, and many feel misunderstood and unsupported in it. This book is here to help support you. When your medical health is in a precarious place, you are filled with fear. You need safety and comfort in a medical system that understands your symptoms and your needs – a system with practitioners who encourage self-advocacy in your healing journey.

I believe in all forms of medicine – we need to integrate all the tools available in the perfect combination to solve the problem. All of these forms are necessary at different points in the healing process. Modern medicine is fast-acting on symptoms that need to be immediately addressed; the ancient systems of medicine (often falling under alternative medicine) and psychotherapy will assist with the deeper roots, but these may take some time to act.

This book comes from a place of wisdom acquired through trauma. It is intended as a guidance system for those who are out of balance. As a clinical psychologist untrained in anything medical, I have been trying to figure out the human body as best as I can to help me guide people to the right places for their healing. This I have done as the universe sent me a dark night of the soul in the form of an autoimmune scare. I have gradually turned myself around, with some setbacks along the way. Perhaps this book will assist you, or provide a starting point if you are completely in the dark. Ultimately, this illness will release once you have dealt with its psychological or metaphysical aspects, and you have transformed the path of your life. In the meantime, support your body through this transformation process in whichever ways feel right for you, but don't get stuck in the supporting the body part – see the greater pathway this is illuminating for you. Your life needs a makeover.

Autoimmune disease is often explained as an overactive immune system that attacks the body. I don't really want to argue with modern medicine here as I understand there are reasons for this being formulated in this manner. However, I believe this requires correction: your body is perfect, and your immune system would never turn against itself. Your body is here to support you in your healing. What your immune system is doing is reacting to the many toxins and pathogens inside it that have accumulated due to the weakened detoxification and prolonged stress that have created a vulnerability to these pathogens. If you are under attack from a virus, your organs may appear to be degrading as a consequence of your immune system being in overdrive. But before you make this assumption, please check for anything else that may be causing this degradation – much of the time there is a source. Many people have autoimmune-like symptoms and don't even know it. My own mother complained for years of a pain in her rib cage – costochondritis. Symptoms such as nerve pain, back pain, seizures, anxiety, depression, headaches, migraines, cysts, hormone imbalances, hair loss, tinnitus, eye floaters, teeth chattering, jaw weakness or tightness, nausea, bleeding gums, tics, spasms, panic attacks, tightness in the chest, tremors, shaking, and being easily upset and triggered, among others, are often ignored but may represent something deeper that needs investigation and support.

As I discuss in Part 2, psychoneuroimmunology speaks to stress being the driver behind illness. Most of the chronic conditions I have seen in my practice are rooted in just this, often piled on to a mountain of childhood trauma. The unpredictability of life today, if we look at factors such as the pandemic, climate change and political instability, leads us to live in a constant state of adrenal dysregulation. Our water is not clean, our food is full of chemicals, and we are living in a 5G microwave oven. Add to that some relationship or financial difficulties, and you have an adrenaline disaster flooding the body. When we have already come from a place of childhood trauma and its consequent adrenal dysregulation, we are not left with much resilience to cope with matters in the present. Our psychology begins the process of wearing away our body.

But working through our psychology alone is not what will reverse this. We need to unwind the damage in the body through detoxification and strengthening, along with addressing the psychological aspects that have driven us to a halt. We need to undo the physiological progression and set ourselves on a different trajectory to health. The body's emotional and physical balance needs many healing elements to re-establish itself. We live in a paradigm in which there isn't a direct cause and effect; there are many causes and many effects. These diseases are developmental: you could start to realise that your illness has been going on for a long time, in different forms – throughout your life, in fact. Often, a timeline of your trauma history, emotional health and physical health is a good place to begin.

 Task

It would be useful right now to draw a timeline of your life traumas, stressful occurrences and health history, and to observe how these may coincide. This could be the start of your investigations. An important question to ask about each of your symptoms is, when did it start?

My story

When I look at where this all began for me, it is far before the time when any of my autoimmune symptoms came about. The symptoms allowed me to notice that something wasn't right about how I was choosing to live my life. My immune system had never been what it should have been – perhaps as a consequence of my traumatic premature birth where my hips were displaced, or of my adrenaline levels due to conflict between my parents, or of having an anxious mother, or of having moved countries twice during childhood. There were probably many traumas and micro-traumas that drove my adrenaline up and my immune system down, and I became a sickly child.

I remember frequenting doctors and taking a string of antibiotics. It was as though I always had flu or some more severe version, like bronchitis. When I look back, I get this sense that I was always sick – or taking a lot of care not to get sick. I remember a stage with lots of UTIs when I was in my twenties.

There was a point of no return, though – at age 26, when my body never felt the same again. It was a difficult relationship, and a series of traumatic experiences, a strict corporate job and a virus that sent me over the edge. I felt terrible chronic fatigue for months. At some point during this time I was admitted to hospital with a very high viral load and a suspicious virus that was never investigated. I got myself back in action with the help of an acupuncturist and lots of juicing. Little did I know that this would affect the next ten years of my life, without my having any idea of the carnage it was gradually wreaking in my system.

On an intuitive level, I was careful about my diet and supported myself through acupuncture, hot yoga and steam rooms. I was managing the fatigue that I took to be a normal part of working life. I did not know that it was not normal to feel this way.

Once you notice your symptoms, a deep psychological process begins, starting with a vacillation between fear and denial. Denial and suppression are important defence mechanisms for those with autoimmune conditions. We are people who bury difficulty deep inside our bodies – we push ourselves, we survive. At this time, much of the fear you are feeling is also a physiological effect of what is happening in the body. Autoimmunity causes the most rampant anxiety. This occurs through various pathways, but it often begins with a viral attack on the vagus nerve, and dysregulated neurotransmitters in the brain.

Those of us who bring illness into our body tend to live in our minds – it's time to get out of your head and into your body and your emotions. Your body feels uncomfortable right now but the only way to begin to heal it is to reconnect with it. This reconnection will help you find your internal guide to healing yourself. Take some distance from the diagnosis and prognosis (if you have these), as they can make you lose hope. The most important companions on your healing journey are hope, patience and motivation (which includes discipline). Your body is telling you that your life can be lived in a better way. Commit to the power of discipline; there is something that gets unlocked inside of us through the reclamation of agency and choice.

This book is here to help you be your own detective and turn yourself around. It is written from a place of experience rather than science. It has three parts. Part 1 explains what autoimmunity is, detailing some of the more common diagnoses, as well as other trauma-driven conditions. Part 2 discusses the causes of autoimmune and other trauma-driven conditions. It is divided into sections, but it is important to recognise that these are all interlinked, just as the mind and body should be considered as one. Part 3 proposes some solutions to the problems you are experiencing. This book is by no means complete in terms of the information it provides. Each of the modalities described in this book can be delved into much more deeply than these limited pages allow. There is also probably so much I don't know that I don't know. This book is what I do know. I wish someone had told me to take care of my immune system when I was younger and taught me how to do this. This book does just that – it helps you understand what your immune system needs to come back online.

What is autoimmunity?

Scientists have defined more than eighty autoimmune conditions. I have listed and discussed the ones that come up frequently in my practice, as well as some prominent other stress- and trauma-related conditions that seem to have a similar causal mechanism to autoimmune conditions. An all-inclusive list probably demands a book of its own and describing these conditions extensively will not be my focus here.

How I understand it is that we all have vulnerabilities in our bodies, and that these are the areas that fail first when we are pushed too hard by trauma and stress. The main areas that are implicated in these conditions are the joints, thyroid, kidneys, liver, lungs, skin and nerves. People are often diagnosed with multiple autoimmune and stress-related conditions; I have seen long lists of these in my practice. Your diagnosis is not your destiny. Perhaps it is worth looking at autoimmune manifestation as a continuum on which each individual crosses over to certain symptoms in a unique order, often based on their genetic predispositions. What I have noticed with my patients and myself is that when you heal, your symptoms generally reverse in the order in which they arrived. In treating autoimmune conditions and other stress- and trauma-related illness, what is important is addressing each individual symptom both physically and emotionally by finding its roots.

Louise Hay has written a book called *You Can Heal Your Life*. I highly recommend this book as part of your journey of healing to introduce you to the emotional meaning of your symptoms until you are in tune enough with that aspect of yourself to begin to decipher your symptoms yourself. Another book you can consult here is Deb Shapiro's *Your Body Speaks Your Mind*. I will touch on these in the discussion that follows.

Chronic fatigue syndrome (CFS)

This is the symptom (or diagnosis) at which most of us begin this journey. CFS is not an autoimmune condition, but it is often a first stop on this road. The main symptoms of CFS are severe and debilitating fatigue, both physical and mental. The fatigue can be persistent or come and go but will have lasted for at least four months before a diagnosis can be made. It is not relieved by rest and is accompanied by a myriad of physical and mental symptoms.

Physical symptoms include painful muscles, joint pain, a sore throat, headaches, dizziness, flu-like symptoms, or difficulty regulating temperature. Mental symptoms include poor short-term memory and concentration; depression is also common. Sufferers often complain of disturbed sleep and that the fatigue is usually worse a day or two after increased mental or physical activity and can then be prolonged. Infections or immunisations may also make it worse. Many people also become completely intolerant of alcohol.

While no single cause of CFS has been identified, there are known triggers. These are often infections, particularly glandular fever caused by the Epstein-Barr virus (EBV), coxsackievirus and cytomegalovirus. A fatigue state may be brought on if you have insufficient rest during an infection, or sometimes if you take fever-suppressant drugs. Less common triggers include major trauma, operations, vaccinations and some pesticides.

The causes of CFS are debated, but as yet no laboratory tests exist to confirm the diagnosis. I believe the reason for this is that it is quite simply driven by a virus. What is known is that it is commonly associated with a respiratory or gastrointestinal viral infection and a resultant abnormality in the immune system, which some see as being in a state of overactivity. This makes sense in terms of the underlying virus the body is fighting.

CFS can have a huge effect, as those who have it are often severely limited in their ability to carry out the normal activities of daily living. Its severity is defined by the degree to which it affects a person's functioning and daily life. This is quite simply mild, moderate or severe. With mild CFS people are mobile, can care for themselves and may be able to work, although they will often need a whole weekend to rest. At the most severe end of the scale, sufferers are unable to do any activity for themselves, may spend most of their time in bed, have severe cognitive problems and can even be wheelchair dependent.

Louise Hay links EBV to pushing yourself beyond your limits due to experiencing yourself as not good enough, draining all your inner support. EBV is understood as the stress virus. In my practice, most of my burnout and chronic fatigue clients experienced the trauma of conditional acceptance in their childhood – that love was conditional upon them performing or being a particular way (displaying certain rewarded qualities) and there not being a sense that they were accepted no matter what they did or who they were.

This leads to frenetic achievement, striving and pleasing behaviours, which undoubtedly result in fatigue.

Fibromyalgia syndrome (FMS)

Fibromyalgia syndrome is a condition characterised by chronic widespread pain and tenderness at specifically defined points in the soft fibrous tissues of the body. Like chronic fatigue syndrome (CFS), it is not classified as an autoimmune condition; however, it resembles many of the symptoms of autoimmune conditions and may have a similar causal pathway.

In FMS, painful stimuli are often felt very intensely (hyperalgesia) and non-painful stimuli, such as brushing, can also be felt as pain (allodynia). It is a newly recognised illness that also features widespread stiffness, deep fatigue, depression, anxiety, sleep disturbance, headaches, migraines, variable bowel habits and diffuse abdominal pain (irritable bowel syndrome), and urinary frequency. It can come and go and is of indeterminate length. The exhaustion may be so draining that it can make it hard to function, either mentally or physically, and there appears to be abnormal sensory processing, which increases the pain experienced. There also appears to be a strong connection to CFS – some experts say the two are simply variations of the same thing – as FMS also has a possible post-viral cause and the two illnesses share many of the same symptoms. It is also said to be found more frequently in patients diagnosed with rheumatoid arthritis (RA) and systemic lupus erythematosus (SLE).

The cause of FMS is not known. It is likely that different people diagnosed with FMS are suffering from the symptoms for different reasons. Some of the suggestions include hyperexcitability of the central nervous system (CNS), alterations in the mechanisms for the perception of pain and interactions with the limbic system, which governs sleep and stress-and immune-regulating systems. The hyperexcitable CNS and limbic system activation indicates a link to psychological trauma. Various symptoms of FMS mimic those of coxsackicvirus.

Interpretations of Louise Hay support the link between FMS and trauma, with possible post-traumatic stress disorder (PTSD) or sexual abuse. According to Deb Shapiro, FMS is a fear showing up as extreme tension due to stress. There is a lowered tolerance to pain, probably due to a dysfunctional sensory system. This says that repressed psychoemotional tension is affecting you to the point that it is distorting your perception, which in turn is lowering your tolerance (or patience), creating a deep inner pain. This is a repressed resistance to your circumstances, a longing to pull back, as your tolerance for what is happening, whether in yourself or in your world, is close to non-existent. This affects your entire nervous system, giving rise to sleep disorders and other ailments. The deep fatigue indicates a longing to give up, an exhaustion from having to cope or carry on beyond your limits. This illness implies a loss of purpose or direction, and a loss of spirit. It is as if the desire to participate and enter life has drained away, leaving you without intention or motivation.

Inflammatory bowel disease (IBD)

In inflammatory bowel disease, it is believed that the immune system attacks the lining of the intestines, causing episodes of diarrhoea, rectal bleeding, urgent bowel movements, abdominal pain, fever and weight loss. Ulcerative colitis and Crohn's disease are the two major forms of IBD. Oral and injected immune-suppressing medicines are typically used to treat IBD.

Ulcerative colitis causes inflammation and ulcers (sores) in your digestive tract. It affects the innermost lining of your large intestine (colon) and rectum. Symptoms usually develop over time, rather than suddenly. It can be debilitating and can sometimes lead to life-threatening complications.

Louise Hay links IBD to overexacting parents, a feeling of oppression or defeat, and a great need for affection. Perhaps the body here has created allergens and sensitivities to various foods it can no longer tolerate as it is overwhelmed by something else going on and that it can no longer tolerate in the emotional background. I believe there is a similar causal aetiology to CFS here, but greater degradation has perhaps taken place in the gut rather than in the liver. Hay links Crohn's disease to fear, worry and not feeling good enough. Worth mentioning here, but not in the same category as IBD, is coeliac disease, a digestive disorder in which your immune system attacks cells of the small intestine when you ingest gluten. On a symbolic level, bread and gluten have been linked to father energy. This is often something to do with not being able to assimilate one's father for various reasons. Bread is grounding and is linked to the root chakra – our roots. It can also be symbolic of a separation from the family. Most people with autoimmune conditions are gluten intolerant, and most have family roots that have been shaky at best. According to Louise Hay, the intestines represent assimilation and absorption – and by this she likely means the circumstances around you.

Endometriosis

Endometriosis is an increasingly common gynaecological condition in which the primary symptom is pelvic pain appearing during or around the menstrual period. It occurs when the tissue that normally lines the uterus (the endometrium) begins to grow outside of the uterus. Part of the endometrium backs up into the fallopian tubes and pelvic cavity, where it sticks to the organs and/or the pelvic wall and continues to function as uterine tissue. The main symptoms are painful periods, heavy periods, pelvic pain, pain on intercourse, ovarian cysts and sometimes bowel symptoms. Often, those with endometriosis have dysregulation in their endocrine system. This is usually due to higher-than-average adrenaline and oestrogen levels. High adrenaline knocks out the immune system, which causes dormant pathogens to come to the surface. High oestrogen could be a sign that the liver is not processing this hormone adequately, perhaps indicating a strained liver.

Louse Hay believes endometriosis is linked to a sense of insecurity, disappointment and frustration. According to Deb Shapiro, from a metaphysical perspective endometriosis can be a fear of bearing children or the consequence of childbirth. This can include the fear of complications and discomfort during pregnancy and even childbirth itself. Endometriosis can carry a deeply hidden fear of dying or suffering in the process of delivery. This can be compounded if the mother had difficulties during birth. A lack of self-love and insecurity may have originated in childhood, often accompanied by self-blame. It may also be a result of rejecting one's femininity and personal power. There may be a deep disappointment in the self, with unresolved sadness and frustration.

Ankylosing spondylitis

Ankylosing spondylitis is an inflammatory disease that, over time, can cause some of the bones in the spine (vertebrae) to fuse. This fusing makes the spine less flexible, can cause a fusion of the joints, and results in a fixed, hunched posture. If the ribs are affected, it can be difficult to breathe deeply. This is a most unpleasant form of arthritis, which predominantly affects young men aged 20 to 40. Craniosacral therapy and physiotherapy are important here to keep the back supple.

Lower back problems, according to Louise Hay, represent a lack of support. They are also associated with the root chakra from yogic and Ayurvedic systems, which represents home, safety and belonging. The few people I have met with this disease have a marked trauma history affecting those themes, and a tendency to be a caregiver to many (often providing the care they may never have received themselves). Typical trauma events that are mentioned by individuals with this diagnosis include birth trauma, abandonment, physical neglect, poor physical bonding and attachment with the mother in early years, malnourishment, feeding difficulties in early years, physical abuse and violent early environments. I imagine a life of living on adrenaline for those who eventually get to this diagnosis. This adrenaline turns off the immune system and invites pathogens to come into action, which then turns the immune system back on – but perhaps not enough to conquer these pathogens. The pathogens specifically target the area (or chakra) that has been weakened over time through the consequences of life trauma.

Rheumatoid arthritis (RA)

Rheumatoid arthritis is a condition that runs in families and has a progressive course, with sufferers sometimes ending up with a crippling disease of many joints. It is known as an autoimmune disease, which is understood as the body attacking its own joints. The immune system produces antibodies that attach to the linings of joints. Immune system cells then attack the joints, causing inflammation, swelling and pain. If untreated, it gradually causes permanent joint damage.

Researchers think the disease may be started by a microbial infection. Sometimes the onset is abrupt and is accompanied by an acute febrile illness that causes swelling and redness in one or more joints. The joints remain painful and swollen after the fever settles, and often further joints get affected. More frequently the onset is insidious, presenting with pain in the small joints of the fingers or toes. These joints swell and become deformed, ending up with the characteristic rheumatoid picture of ulnar deviation. Other joints, commonly shoulders, knees, ankles and elbows, are also affected. The joints grow increasingly painful and inflexible, which severely restricts movement and expression.

Louise Hay links RA to a deep criticism of authority and feeling very put upon. According to Deb Shapiro, the body–mind symptoms of RA indicate that there may be repressed anger. Many people with this condition have previously been very active, such as athletes who can channel their energy into sport, but this does not necessarily resolve the underlying issue – when they retire, they have nowhere to put those angry feelings. Emotions are very involved here, especially the expression of love. A way to healing this is finding that expression.

Psoriasis

In psoriasis, immune system blood cells called T-cells collect in the skin. This immune system activity stimulates skin cells to reproduce rapidly, producing silvery, scaly plaques on the skin, which result in symptoms such as itchiness, cracked, dry skin, skin pain, nails that are pitted or crumble, and joint pain.

At first, red bumps grow on the skin, and then scales form on top of these. The surface scales might shed easily, but the scales beneath may then stick together. If scratched, the scales may tear away from the skin, causing it to bleed. As the rash continues to grow, lesions may form. The causes are believed to be emotional stress, streptococcal or other infections that affect the immune system, certain prescription medications like lithium and beta blockers, and cold weather (reduced exposure to sunlight and humidity).

Louise Hay links psoriasis to a fear of being hurt, deadening the senses, and refusing to accept responsibility for one's own feelings.

Hashimoto's thyroiditis

Hashimoto's thyroiditis is defined as an autoimmune disease in which the immune system turns against the thyroid gland. The thyroid gland, a small gland behind the trachea in the neck, influences the chemistry of your whole body and can thus cause a wide array of symptoms. The thyroid produces hormones for growth, cell regeneration and repair; it maintains both metabolism (including heart rate and how quickly your body uses calories from the foods you eat) and oxygen consumption.

Symptoms can include fatigue, pain in muscles and joints, increased sensitivity to cold, a puffy face, hair loss, enlargement

Due to its widespread effect on the body, it can create many symptoms. It usually starts with joint pain, especially in the small joints of the hands and feet, which may flit from one set of joints to another. Skin rashes are also common. Patients often have fever, malaise, weight loss and fatigue. Lymph glands in the neck and other parts of the body are often tender and swollen, and muscles may ache and be tender to touch. Treatment often requires daily oral prednisone, a steroid that reduces immune system function.

Those presenting in my practice with lupus have an extensive trauma history, starting from a young age. If we look at something like lupus on the chakra system, we can imagine that there is a disruption in balance in all the chakras. Louise Hay links lupus to giving up, the belief that it is better to die than to stand up for yourself.

Sjögren's syndrome

Sjögren's (SHOW-grins) syndrome is a disorder of the immune system identified by its two most common symptoms – dry eyes and a dry mouth. Your eyes might burn, itch or feel gritty, as if there is sand in them. Your mouth may feel like it is full of cotton wool, making it difficult to swallow or speak. The condition often accompanies other immune system disorders, such as RA and lupus.

In Sjögren's syndrome, the mucous membranes and moisture-secreting glands of your eyes and mouth are usually affected first, resulting in decreased tears and saliva. Some people with Sjögren's syndrome also have one or more of the following: joint pain, swelling and stiffness, swollen salivary glands (particularly the set located behind your jaw and in front of your ears), skin rashes or dry skin, vaginal dryness, a persistent dry cough and prolonged fatigue. In Sjögren's syndrome, it is believed that your immune system first targets the glands that make tears and saliva. But it can also damage other parts of your body, such as the joints, thyroid, kidneys, liver, lungs, skin and nerves.

Guillain-Barré syndrome and chronic inflammatory demyelinating polyneuropathy

In these autoimmune conditions, the immune system attacks the nerves that govern the muscles in the legs, and occasionally the arms and upper torso. Severe weakness often results. The main form of treatment for Guillain-Barré syndrome involves filtering the blood via a process known as plasmapheresis. Chronic inflammatory demyelinating polyneuropathy is similar to Guillain-Barré in that the immune system also attacks the nerves, but symptoms last much longer. If the condition is not identified and treated early, about 30 per cent of patients risk becoming wheelchair-bound. Metaphysically, nerves represent communication; they are receptive reporters. Louise Hay ascribes neuralgia to punishment for guilt, and anguish about communication.

Multiple sclerosis (MS)

A complex illness, multiple sclerosis affects people in many different ways. It is known as an autoimmune disease as the immune system appears to attack the myelin sheath surrounding the nerves, leading to sclerosis and the inability of the nerves to communicate fully, but there are differing theories for this and nothing conclusive. The effects of MS depend on the extent of the nerve damage that takes place. Symptoms include numbness, nerve pain, difficulties with balance and moving, eyesight problems, deep exhaustion, poor coordination, weakness and muscle spasms. These issues vary in duration and severity, making a clear prognosis difficult. Typically, various medicines that suppress the immune system are used to treat MS.

Emotional stress plays a big role in the occurrence of MS episodes, with episodes being triggered after periods of intense stress. This may apply to the other conditions I discuss here too, but in MS there is quite a marked activation of symptoms. Although stress is an obvious cause, research is also suggesting that there are other, more intricate, causes. There may be difficulties in the vascular system, specifically the return of blood from the brain to the heart. Metaphysically, this may be ascribed to difficulties with receiving, or perhaps a disconnection between the brain and heart, where there is too much focus on thinking and not enough on feeling.

Diabetes

Diabetes occurs when there is not enough insulin in the body to cope with the incoming glucose (as in type 2 diabetes), or if the pancreas fails to produce any insulin (as in type 1 diabetes). Sugar accumulates in the blood and is released in the urine, rather than being transformed into energy. This can lead to a drop in energy and may be fatal if left unattended. It is the sixth most common cause of death, and the second most common cause of blindness.

Insulin has to be provided, either through a change in diet or through insulin injections, depending on the type of diabetes. The signs of diabetes are often subtle, but they can become severe. They include extreme thirst, increased hunger, dry mouth, upset stomach and vomiting, frequent urination, unexplained weight loss, fatigue, blurry vision, laboured breathing, mood changes, infections of the skin, urinary tract or vagina, and bedwetting. Type 1 diabetes can develop when a virus, for example, causes your immune system to attack your pancreas. This type of diabetes leaves autoantibodies, which are traces of this attack.

Louise Hay links diabetes to a longing for what might have been, a great need to control, deep sorrow, and no sweetness left in life. According to Deb Shapiro, just as diabetics cannot integrate or use the sugar in the food they eat, so it is hard for them to integrate or accept love. Diabetes is particularly related to feeling either a lack or an overabundance of sweetness in your life. This may form through loss or loneliness. Children can develop diabetes at a time of parental conflict, such as divorce or death, feeling that they are the cause of the loss, or that the parent no longer loves them, or due to a smothering, excessively adoring parent. Adult diabetes can occur during times when you feel undernourished emotionally. It also occurs in connection with obesity, which is often linked to a loss of love or fear of intimacy; it shows the link between overeating to make up for a lack of love and an inability to receive love. Stress can also have an isolating effect: you feel that no one really cares, or you become unable to absorb any love that is available, losing your sense of emotional balance.

It is hard to be independent if you have a constant dependence on insulin. This creates a dependence on the home – diabetic children may live at home for longer than others – and a difficulty in making personal relationships last. There is also resentment: a desire to be loved but not to have to love, to be cared for without having to give. When the inner sweetness passes straight through and leaves in the urine, it causes a sadness or sense of loss. People with diabetes often feel emotionally isolated, unable to give of themselves. Learning to love yourself and finding the right balance of give and take is essential.

Long COVID and the vaccine

As research develops, trends point to long COVID being an activation of dormant co-viruses in the system that leave lingering effects. This will perhaps be clarified in the years to come. It makes sense, however, that COVID-19 potentially weakens the immune system, allowing these viruses to come to prominence. EBV, coxsackievirus, human papilloma virus (HPV) and the various herpes viruses, among others, have been mentioned as being activated in this way.

Long COVID then resembles an autoimmune condition, with symptoms such as joint pain, headaches, nerve pain, anxiety and others. The vaccine may also have the quality of awakening dormant viruses in the system, and we have seen it launch an autoimmune cascade in some people, although this is all still very speculative at this time. This, in the context of the trauma of the pandemic, has led to adrenal dysregulation and the consequent hijacking of the immune system, making it very difficult for the co-occurring viruses to be fought off effectively. Perhaps this is the explanation for the lingering effects some people are experiencing? The contents of this book can assist you here. Treat yourself as though you are at the beginning of an autoimmune condition, following the guidance in this book that resonates with you. Be gentle with yourself and your symptoms will reverse in the order in which they arrived. These conditions don't have to be permanent.

Psychiatric conditions

Many diseases that were initially considered to be unrelated to autoimmunity are now being re-explored as autoimmune-related, especially in the field of psychiatry. These include major depressive disorder (MDD), schizophrenia, Parkinson's disease, Alzheimer's disease and anxiety. The comorbidity between autoimmune conditions and mental and mood disorders, such as MDD, anxiety, schizophrenia and bipolar disorder, has become apparent in the past two decades. You have a higher risk of developing clinical depression or mood disorders if you have been diagnosed with an autoimmune condition; all the autoimmune patients I have in my practice suffer from anxiety and at least occasional depression. Research indicates that neurological involvement has been found in many autoimmune diseases, with psychiatric abnormalities such as anxiety, depression, psychosis and cognitive dysfunction.

While there is certainly an argument that the burden of having an autoimmune condition could contribute to MDD, researchers suggest that depression and anxiety symptoms could be a result of autoimmune mechanisms and the resulting inflammation in the nervous system. Even postpartum depression suggests an autoimmune activity that comes into existence through the trauma of birth. PMS is a manifestation of this response, in that a woman's immune system is strained during this time and pathogen activation may bring the mood symptoms about.

༄༅

Diagnosing and treating autoimmune and other trauma-driven conditions

The main means of diagnosing autoimmune and other trauma-driven conditions medically depends on the condition. Blood testing determines the present homeostatic balance in the body. I recommend this as a starting point in your healing journey. It is good to know what is happening right now and have this on paper to see. Check your thyroid, oestrogen, progesterone, testosterone, serotonin, vitamin D, magnesium, iron and vitamin B12 levels as a start; in addition, test for coxsackievirus, EBV, *Helicobacter pylori* and cytomegalovirus, and anything else your integrative medicine doctor may recommend. BioScan and other such methods (discussed later) can also provide a picture of what is going on internally.

Specifically, RA investigations could include blood tests for rheumatoid factor, anti-CCP antibodies and erythrocyte sedimentation rate (ESR) to determine presence of inflammatory mediators; an X-ray to identify the extent of damage to the joints; an MRI to determine the severity of the condition; and arthrocentesis, a procedure during which a sterile needle is used to withdraw joint fluid to determine the cause of symptoms. Hashimoto's typically entails a series of thyroid-specific blood tests and a thyroid ultrasound. Lupus diagnosis includes a full blood count to check the count of platelets and red blood cells, and an ESR test as well. In this test, the time taken for red blood cells to settle at the bottom of a test tube is faster than normal in people with lupus. Lupus diagnosis also involves urine analysis as high protein and red blood cell levels might indicate kidney damage, an antinuclear antibody test, a skin biopsy and a kidney biopsy.

Alternative diagnostic methods may be of assistance in pinpointing specific symptoms and imbalances. Iridology is an alternative medicine technique whose proponents claim that the patterns, colours and other characteristics of the iris can be examined to determine information about a patient's systemic health. Like markings on a map, the iris can reveal physiological and psychological conditions, constitutional strengths and weaknesses, nutritional deficiencies, the challenges of various organs, areas of inflammation, injury or degeneration, and the overall integrity of the body. Through iridology, you can get an understanding of your past, present and potential future health conditions by assessing the various body systems. Your inherited tendencies compounded by toxic accumulations in various parts of your body are also revealed. The iris contains many nerve endings that are connected to the optic nerve, the base of the brain and all the bodily tissues. Hence, the neural circuitry of the eye can express the continuity of the body, an integrated unit composed of various cells that all communicate with the irises about their overall wellness.

Kinesiology is a form of therapy that uses muscle monitoring (body feedback) to look at imbalances that may be causing disease in the body. It aims to detect and correct imbalances that may relate to stress, nutrition or minor injuries. The kinesiology approach examines 'unresolved stress reactions' in a person and provides techniques intended to help the body's natural healing process. Ayurveda diagnoses illness through eight different areas: Nadi (pulse), Mootra (urine), Mala (stool), Jihva (tongue), Shabda (speech), Sparsha (touch), Druk (vision) and Aakruti (appearance).

Traditional Chinese medicine (TCM) inspects a person's spirit, complexion, body shape, posture, tongue and pulse to determine what is happening in the five organ systems based on the presenting symptoms. The tongue is very important in these systems, and I have found myself studying my tongue in the mirror as an effective method of observing my health over time. The tongue has various features that indicate aspects of different bodily functions. For example, the colour of the tongue body may indicate the state of the blood, organs and *qi* (life force). Tongue body features such as teeth marks, indicating that the tongue rests against the teeth, may be a sign of inflammation or a digestive disorder that is typical of autoimmune conditions. The tongue coating may reveal the state of organs, and the thickness of this coating may indicate an imbalance in digestion or be associated with allergic disorders and autoimmune diseases.

While the causes of autoimmune conditions are controversial, there seem to be many facets that contribute to their development, such as genetic predisposition, environmental triggers and psychosocial stress. At a causal level they all seem to be a manifestation of an adrenal, emotional, toxin and pathogen overload in your system. There is strong evidence that traumatic experiences such as adverse childhood events (ACEs) and prolonged stress may contribute to the development of autoimmunity. Common characteristics observed among the various types of autoimmunity include increased intestinal permeability, chronic inflammation, the presence of chronic infections, a dysregulated hypothalamic-pituitary-adrenal (HPA) axis, mitochondrial dysfunction and microbiome imbalance. Symptoms can manifest as chronic fatigue, allergies, psychiatric and mood disorders, pain, rashes, gastrointestinal (GI) distress, poor cognition and more. Listening to my patients' symptoms triggers me into thinking that we all seem to have the same thing, in different manifestations. I am behind the thinking that these are all pathogen-driven, and it is worth asking how the pathogen came to be there – which leads me to question how stress and trauma disrupt the body's natural microbiome and homeostatic balance.

Currently, biologics and immunosuppressant drugs are the primary treatment tools for autoimmune disorders, along with non-steroidal anti-inflammatory drugs, steroids and antidepressants. When you take corticosteroids for inflammatory diseases like RA or asthma, the adrenal glands balance the body by reducing their production of cortisol. However, immunosuppressant and biologic medications designed to resemble antibodies, receptors and other immunological factors can result in an immune-compromised state, putting you at risk for serious infections or immune-related illnesses. Although existing biologics approaches show evidence of producing positive treatment outcomes in some individuals, the increased risks of infection, malignancy and cardiovascular conditions, as well as contradictory results in efficacy studies, have prompted interest in exploring other treatment approaches.

The aim of some of these treatments is to suppress an overactive immune system. But I don't think enough is being asked about why the immune system is overactive. Would your immune system really attack your body? Our bodies are for us surviving, not against us. We have instincts that make us fear dangers like heights and snakes for our own survival. Surely this intelligent design would not build in an out-of-control immune system?

According to Deb Shapiro, anyone with an autoimmune or trauma-driven condition should ask themselves the following questions, which require a bit of digging past the denial in which we usually operate from day to day:

- How have you become an enemy to yourself?
- To what extent do you allow others to influence you in denying your own thoughts or feelings?
- Do you feel as if you are not really valid?
- Do you think you don't have needs?
- Are you carrying guilt, shame or blame from the past that is wearing away your self-esteem or self-respect?
- Do you have an underlying dislike or hatred of yourself?
- Do you spend your time helping others but refusing help yourself?
- Are you overly critical of yourself?
- Do you constantly put yourself down?
- Is someone else wearing away at you, corroding your sense of worth?
- Have you lost your ability to discriminate?
- Do you let others determine what you think or feel?

PART 2

What causes autoimmune and other trauma-driven conditions?

THERE ARE VARIOUS streams of thinking on the cause of autoimmune conditions. Each of the practitioners I have seen has tended to be swayed by a specific dominant camp. It is certainly clear, however, that a multitude of factors is at play.

Firstly, *biomedical causes*: these include factors such as genetic predisposition; viruses, bacteria or other pathogens; and medications, accidents or injuries that may activate or exacerbate an autoimmune condition.

Next are *psychosomatic causes*, the camp where I dominantly sit in my practice. Here, the thinking is that autoimmune conditions are caused by all kinds of stress and psychological trauma and their effects on us, including negative thoughts, false beliefs and the personality manifestations of trauma. These include being out of balance with our authentic selves and needs – for example, we are working too hard at the expense of love and connection; or we are working in an environment that is not in line with our soul's true calling; or perhaps we are in a relationship that is sapping our life force. This in turn creates energy blockages in the body that, over time, manifest in illness such as autoimmunity.

I have already touched on *environmental causes* in the introduction, including pollution, the dysregulation of the earth's microbiome and our compromised water supply, as well as the changing interaction between men and women in society. In a talk called 'Authenticity can heal trauma', physician Gabor Maté states that 'we are the only species that creates environments that are destructive to our own species'. Our family environment and country of residence contribute heavily here, too.

 Task

Important to note is the wide net of interaction between all these factors, the interconnection between body and mind, and internal and external systems that are out of balance. Perhaps, before we dive into the details of the causal factors, you can note down what you think is driving your specific condition.

Stress

Stress is any physiological event, external or internal, that demands that the body adapt to it. There is a basic tension in our everyday life based on the continued need to achieve certain goals to survive. The most elemental needs include food, drink, shelter and procreation. Thereafter, our basic 'needs' become shaped by our cultural expectations, which are directly related to and shaped by the complexity of our culture itself.

When we were hunter-gatherers on the African plains, these needs were pretty simple. As we've moved to more complex models of cultural organisation, our basic needs have reflected that complexity, and the definition of stress has broadened accordingly. Every cultural and technological advance brings new, unique stressors and demands new kinds of problem solving and adaptation. Moving from simplicity to complexity in any state of life will do this. It has taken less than a century for long-distance communication to evolve from the operator-assisted phone call to smartphones and instant international communication. Every 'labour-saving' device comes at the price of effortful new learning and, if you wish, stress. Progress is achieved through this adaptive process.

In a society that commends hard work, many believe that if life is too easy, we're not doing enough. We believe that the harder we work, and the longer we persist, the more we will be celebrated for our resilience and strength. Perhaps we need to change this narrative about how life should unfold, with our focus rather being on flow. This means being in touch with our inner guide rather than looking to society for what we should do – and listening to our bodies and their needs. To flow means to surrender, soften, allow and accept that life is forever changing. We may not be able to control everything around us, but we can control how we react to it.

Try to remember a recent situation in which you faced a specific stress in your life – a broken relationship, a fight with your significant other, a confrontation at work, or the sudden decline in your investment as the stock market tanked, for example. Think back to how you physically felt in your body, what the common theme of your thoughts was, how well (or badly) you slept, and which unpleasant physical sensations you experienced. Did you feel in control, or relatively helpless? Was there anger, or a touch of anxiety or panic? Did you have any bowel symptoms (bloating, indigestion, cramps), heartburn or palpitations? Did you have trouble sleeping, perhaps waking with racing thoughts that repeated and couldn't be shut down?

Did thinking about these things now bring up any of the same symptoms and feelings in your body? All of these common symptoms are typical of the effect of 'little traumas' in our lives – conflicted events over which we had no control, leading to a mixture of arousal and freeze states. This phenomenon is characterised by chronic arousal, sleep disturbance, obsessive persistence, distraction and inattentiveness. Sometimes there are even somatic sensations, most commonly myofascial pain around the neck, bruxism (grinding the teeth), bowel symptoms and fatigue. What you are dealing with is a relatively small but well-defined 'dissociation capsule' that keeps interrupting your present moment and clouding your mind. Stress in the face of helplessness becomes trauma, as far as the brain is concerned.

Stress may also be what we attract into our lives as a consequence of trauma – it is, to some extent, based on our patterns, our level of autonomic nervous system (ANS) dysregulation (which often invites chaos into our lives through the impulsivity and lack of memory and attention that dysregulation causes) and our choices in life. It is also a part of daily life that we need to accept, and many stressors are shared on various levels by most of humanity. Some stress is healthy and motivational – it accelerates us towards our goals. Other stress can easily fall into the category of trauma.

Our response to stress is very important to our health. We turn our stress response on through inadequate sleep, trauma and emotional experiences/exposures, mental exertion and blood sugar imbalances.

The field of medicine called psychoneuroimmunology looks at the link between stress and the immune system. It is a study of the relationship between immunity, the endocrine system, and the central and peripheral nervous system. There are three major components of this model: the psychological component, the neurological component and the immunological component. In this field, the long-standing separation of body and mind dissolves and we see that our emotional states affect our health. Chronic stress or shock trauma can have health repercussions as adrenaline shuts down our immune system. Fight-or-flight mode (survival mode) is not a mode of functioning that allows for the regeneration of the body. The idea that a cheery disposition and positive outlook on life can stave off illness is an old wives' tale that may yet have some merit. In alternative circles, this has been explained for many years by authors such as Louise Hay (*You Can Heal Your Life*), Caroline Myss (*Anatomy of the Spirit*) and Anodea Judith (*Eastern Body, Western Mind*) who speak about how the body manifests the disturbances of the psyche. Examples of the mind–body connection in research include bereavement (stories of people dying soon after the deaths of their partners); how the gut responds to stressful life events; in cases of HIV, how elevated stress and diminished social support accelerate the progression of infection; how psoriasis, eczema and asthma are all known to have psychological aspects; and how our stress levels affect wound healing.

If you want to heal, you need to consider your psychology. Many of the autoimmune clients in my practice cannot list what they enjoy in life. You need to start doing what brings you joy. For example, find a way to make work play so that you don't feel strained by it. In fact, find a way to make everything play. Once it becomes play, it becomes effortless. If you are bored, walk away from what you are doing for a while and come back to it, as boredom can also elicit stress. This can be difficult for most of us. So, let's rather think of maximising joy so that the balance sheet of life leans more towards joyous events than to restrictions and obligations.

You can't heal in the environment that broke you. You may need to find a new path, even though doing so may require energy you don't have right now. As a first step to healing, this may require gathering the energy you have and putting yourself in as comfortable a space as you possibly can. It may mean letting go of certain friends and, as much as it hurts, perhaps also creating the right proximity from certain family members – and finding a place of work where you can feel valued and full of purpose, and express your creativity. You need to feel safe and start to let your guard down so that your adrenal glands can start letting go of leading your life. This will allow your delicate immune system can begin to come back online.

Surfers are known for being chilled. This, I figured out, is due to a well-practised ability to be present. During a surf lesson in Sri Lanka, my instructor said something really valuable to me: 'When you do things with stress, you make them much harder.' He wanted me to stop overthinking the action of getting onto the board and just to stand up gently as I looked ahead. I found myself gripping the board, or pre-empting falling off in my mind. When, finally, I became present and relaxed, and stopped fearing the inevitable

– falling into the water – it suddenly seemed to all go well, and I came to enjoy it more. There is something very valuable about being present and bringing yourself internally to peace. Surfing, like life, requires you to just look ahead and put one foot in front of the other, without overthinking it. We only fall off the board, or off our path in life, when we get caught up in our heads.

 Task

Make a list of all the stressors, frustrations, 'stuckness' and boredom you are facing in your life – all those things you are 'tolerating' that you have moved into the background using your very effective defence mechanisms. For each one, attempt to write down a solution for getting you back in motion (or out of that freeze response).

Trauma

The next natural place to go from stress is trauma – and by this, I mean psychological trauma. Chronic stress and trauma ultimately have the same effect on our bodies. According to Peter Levine, trauma is the physiological and emotional imprint created by anything that is too much or too soon for the nervous system to handle. Trauma lies in those events that overwhelm our ability to cope. We feel helpless and powerless in these events.

Trauma is also a subjective experience, so what I perceive as traumatic may not be what you experience in that way. What is important is that trauma launches the fight, flight, freeze or fawn response in the system – words I am sure you are familiar with by now. As a consequence of these responses, especially in the case of

43

a freeze response, certain emotions become locked into the system. Body sensations and beliefs become locked in, too. As a mentor of mine used to say, it is like a 'blocked irrigation system: information that could not discharge through the normal act of release in a trauma-activating event'.

Because life is filled with traumatic events for all of us, to varying degrees, we can see how, as the years go by, we could lose our childlike essence and become stuck and inflexible. Working through our trauma brings us back to spontaneity and wholeness. We need to get to a place where we have unconditional love for ourselves, act assertively, play comfortably, harness creativity, and live spontaneously.

Psychological trauma can be acute or shock trauma (a sudden event such as a car accident or a robbery), developmental trauma (having a critical or abusive parent, for example) or relational trauma (such as the ending of a relationship). Developmental trauma is trauma that happens during our childhood years and affects how we develop; this includes initial attachment, which sets the foundation of our adrenal regulatory system. The single biggest influence on the behaviour of men and women is the way they were parented. This is also an important predisposing factor to autoimmune conditions.

No one has a greater impact on our self-esteem, world view, beliefs, values, emotional intelligence, the way we handle life and relationships, and the formation of our immune system (through the action on our adrenals) than our caregivers or parents. They teach and model tolerance, love, respect and compassion. A person who is loved as a child is likely to have the capacity for love and compassion as an adult. A person who has structure and comfortable discipline growing up is likely to have self-discipline as an adult. A child who is valued and respected is likely to grow into an adult who respects and values others. Developmental trauma can also take place through teachers, siblings, peers and other adults who are present while we are growing up.

Trauma, then, can be any event that overextends an individual's ability to cope and launches the fight, flight, freeze or fawn response as a survival strategy – responses that all involve the adrenals to some degree. The freeze and fawn responses can be likened to dissociation – the mental process of disconnecting from your thoughts, feelings, memories, or sense of identity. It is a state of being zoned out and shut off. If you had a highly critical parent or were neglected in childhood, freeze or fawn were probably useful to be able to escape the situation while staying physically present in it: as children, we often don't have the means to escape situations physically. Our survival is dependent on our connection to our caregivers.

In trauma, body-based memories are stored as being in the present – even though the traumatic event is in the past – through the imprinting in memory of the sensory and motor patterns of the undischarged freeze response. This storage of 'false' body memories plagues the trauma survivor in the form of intrusive memories, or flashbacks. Post-traumatic memories contain not only the explicit, declarative content and meaning of the event, but also the sensory experiences – smells, images, sounds and body sensations that emerge in the form of sensory symptoms or unconscious movements such as tics.

Humans respond to threats in a similar way to other mammals. When your nervous system becomes overwhelmed and threatened by an unexpected, unwanted stimulus, your body innately and automatically takes certain sequential biological steps as the organism goes into survival mode to regulate the nervous system and rebalance the body. It is the ANS that is responsible for this self-regulation, acting as a control system and prompting the body to return to normalcy. All animals have a natural ability to shake off traumatic experiences. Humans suppress this due to social pressure and the development of the logical brain. The difference between the way in which humans and animals experience threats lies in our utilisation of the many assets of the left brain, which, although vital to our existence, can heighten trauma. This inability to let go is not a cognitive decision, as many trauma victims do not even remember their traumatic experience.

Yet, as Rothschild states in *The Body Remembers*, whether the consciousness chooses to remember and acknowledge the trauma or not, the body remembers. The effects of the experience can remain trapped in the body, embedded in the nervous system as pent-up survival energy, which causes the blockages responsible for the mental, emotional and physical distresses. For as long as the memory of the event is trapped in the body, it will continue to wreak havoc on physical, mental and spiritual health. It is evident that trauma has a significant impact on a person's mental and emotional well-being, but it is less known that traumatic events are physically stored in the human body. So, traditional talk psychotherapy is not always successful at treating trauma, and when it is successful, the recovery is often temporary and unsustainable if it does not include the physical body. Some patients can, and often do, become retraumatised when they verbally and cognitively relate the traumatic experiences in their past.

Trauma energy is often unintegrated, fragmented and very highly charged: your life becomes a bit like walking through a minefield. When your nervous system becomes highly activated, it can sweep you away. The energy has a magnetic pull – hence the term 'vortex' – that takes you out of an integrated sense of self.

 Task

If you are feeling this way at the moment, please put your bare feet firmly on the ground, focusing on moving this trauma energy down your legs and into the ground, feeling rooted on the earth. Please do this regularly if you feel overwhelmed while reading this book.

Stress, trauma and the body–mind connection

In *The Trauma Spectrum: Hidden Wounds and Human Resiliency*, Robert Scaer writes about stress, trauma and the body–mind connection. Much of what I have written below is a summary of this work.

Trauma and stress may result in much unexpressed (suppressed) emotion. These unexpressed emotions hang about in our nervous, muscular, glandular and digestive systems, and/or in other vital body organs, as buried emotions. They remain buried in body organs and systems until we release them by feeling, expressing and venting them. Negative emotions such as fear, anxiety, negativity, frustration and depression cause chemical reactions in the body that are very different from the chemicals released when you feel positive emotions such as happiness, contentment, love and acceptance.

Emotions that are buried continuously and persistently for a prolonged time can cause both medical and psychological conditions, especially autoimmune conditions, which are a mix of these. They can also cause cancer, arthritis, chronic fatigue, digestive

47

disorders, bowel problems and neuropsychic problems. People bury emotions to protect themselves from embarrassing, painful and difficult-to-manage situations at the time of their occurrence. The energy used to bury the repressed emotion can drain the psychic system, creating fatigue, a sense of vulnerability and low self-confidence. Repressed emotions can also control people's behaviour and reactions to past, present and future events. When emotions are blocked in the human psyche they keep on popping up, knowingly and unknowingly – often when triggered by associations in the outside environment. The person affected has to work very hard to keep the blocked emotions stuffed down in the psyche and expends a lot of energy doing so.

The emotional impact of this has been physically investigated. It has been found that the brain can, unfortunately, literally be injured and its function physically impaired because of negative life experiences, stress and emotional trauma. Severe negative life experiences cause shrinkage in the brain and loss of neurons, specifically in the memory centres of the brain. The infant who does not experience the closeness of the maternal–infant bond suffers shrinkage of a crucial area of the brain that regulates the emotional brain and autonomic nervous system. If the brain as the control centre can be affected in this way, we can assume that this has a cascading effect on the other areas of the body. Early in life, the HPA axis is still developing; exposure to trauma during childhood is thought to have profound effects on HPA axis regulation.

The hypothalamus is a small, complex brain centre in the midline base of the brain, directly above the master endocrine gland, the pituitary gland. It has numerous functions, including control of body temperature, hunger, thirst, fatigue, sleep and the sleep/wake cycle. One of its most important functions is stimulating the pituitary gland to release pre-hormones that trigger the release of hormones from the endocrine glands – the thyroid gland, parathyroid gland, adrenal cortex, ovaries and testes. Homeostasis requires optimal balance of all these functions. When we are in adrenal overload, we disrupt all the functions that the hypothalamus controls. This combination of effects sets the stage for all the symptoms that present in autoimmune conditions.

The HPA axis connects our emotions to our physical parts. It is a complex set of feedback interactions that is central to homeostasis, stress responses, energy metabolism and neuropsychiatric function. Stressful stimuli are first sensed by a part of the limbic system called the amygdala, which goes on to activate the HPA axis. In a normal response to stress, there is a negative feedback mechanism to turn the HPA axis off when there is no longer a threat. Trauma, however, disrupts the negative feedback mechanisms of the HPA axis, so that the body is in a chronic state of arousal – it becomes stuck here. This chronic arousal state suppresses the hippocampus, preventing the formation of explicit memory, thus trapping traumatic memories in the implicit system. This is what ultimately goes haywire in PTSD.

The implicit memory system could be called the unconscious mind. Implicit memory allows you to perform actions without needing to consciously recall how to do them, while explicit memory allows you to bring information into conscious awareness. An implicit memory is something like knowing how to ride a bicycle. By storing traumatic memory in this system, we may be creating some difficulties for ourselves. If we have a car accident, it becomes imprinted as cars being dangerous in that implicit system, which could result in anxiety every time we enter a car or attempt to drive as we associatively activate that unconscious memory in the present moment. If this trauma is not processed, the emotions remain trapped and any triggers or associations can reactivate the defensive fight, flight and freeze response. It works like a faulty alarm system; the amygdala goes into overdrive and cannot distinguish between past and present. This is how flashbacks operate. You can't just forget trauma – it's wired into the brain and the logical mind can't change it.

The diseases of trauma are caused by a much more complex, fixed change in specific brain functions. They can't be cured by removing an environmental stimulus. They are based on corrupted procedural memory systems in an altered brain. The causes of these conditions are diverse, based on the shifting, unstable state of the brain and ANS. After trauma, you experience the world with a different nervous system – you are stuck on either your accelerator or your brakes. The sensations of the fight, flight and freeze response stored in your nervous system result in adrenaline being on all the time. Cortisol levels that are too high or too low lead to an underactive immune system and insufficient or defective inflammation to protect us against viruses, infections and other pathogens.

The spectrum of what can happen to the body in stress and trauma is broad and deep. The physical harm to organs and tissues is secondary to elevated cortisol, and includes elevated blood sugar (diabetes), elevated serum lipids (atherosclerosis), elevated stomach acid (peptic ulcers), osteoporosis, elevated blood volume (hypertension), and depressed immune function (opportunistic infections and cancer). Psychological stress and psychoemotional trauma can severely compromise the immune system, leading to an increased risk of chronic infections and a disrupted gut biome: gut dysbiosis. Psychosocial stress increases inflammatory cytokines (a type of cytokine or signalling molecule that is secreted from immune cells and certain other cell types that promotes inflammation), oxidative stress (an imbalance of free radicals and antioxidants in the body, which can lead to cell and tissue damage) and glutamate excitotoxicity (excessive glutamate levels resulting in nerve cell damage). This results in the inhibition of effective digestion and nutrient absorption, and contributes to HPA axis dysfunction. Stress has been found to increase intestinal permeability, which can lead to food sensitivities and inflammation due to gut–blood transepithelial bacterial translocation – more commonly known as 'leaky gut syndrome'.

These inflictions are hallmark characteristics of patients with autoimmune disease. They are specific to an individual hormone rather than a locked-in change in the brain, and they depend upon the continued input of stress to the limbic brain by external, environmental influences. They will persist for as long as the stress continues. If stress proceeds to helplessness, however, the physiology changes from a cortisol endocrine reaction to an autonomic or freeze syndrome. This is when autoimmune conditions begin to manifest. The HPA axis controls the body's inflammatory response. The persistent arousal of the stress response system leaves the body and brain unable to distinguish past from present and takes out the immune system through the mechanism of inflammation. When stress is on overload, our levels of inflammation go up – and inflammation is our pathway to chronic illness, as the body does not heal and rejuvenate in an environment of high inflammation. It should come as no surprise, then, that the abnormal ways in which the brain functions as a result of stress and trauma could 'damage' the body.

Endocrinologist Hans Selye, who did pioneering work in researching stress, actually believed that some stress has a positive effect – the variant of stress that he called eustress, or 'good' stress. Nevertheless, stress does activate the HPA axis, the result being the body's exposure to elevated levels of serum cortisol, which has specific effects on the brain and the body if prolonged. Cortisol causes shrinkage, or atrophy, of the hippocampus. This can cause sleep disturbance and disrupted baseline arousal. A lack of sleep affects the body's ability to rejuvenate itself. From then on, the brain's response is determined by the intensity and severity of the stress and its escalating nature. Cortisol acts as a modulator of the immune system. In high amounts, it suppresses the immune system. Suppression of the immune system makes the body more prone to opportunistic infections by bacteria and viruses that aren't normally very infectious. This is why cold sores are common in people who are stressed, for example.

Good examples of a physical complaint caused by an emotional experience are disorders of the function of the intestinal tract. We've known for a long time that the intestinal tract seems to be sensitive to emotional conflicts and stress, and the gut has often been called our 'second brain'. These 'emotional' gut disorders are associated with abnormal contraction of the gut and impaired sphincters, which are controlled by the brain. The intestines are packed with their own neurons, which actively send messages to the brain that may affect systems of consciousness and memory. So, the body also affects our state of consciousness, the brain itself. This is a constant feedback loop.

These examples only begin to touch on the complexity of the brain–body interface. Cancer, autoimmune conditions of the joints or the intestines, and neurodegenerative diseases have been traced to negative early experiences. These experiences can trigger a lifelong tendency towards inflammation, undermine the immune system and impair or excessively activate the body's stress response mechanisms.

In a study of individuals who died suddenly and inexplicably, all were found to have been faced with inescapable conflict. All their options had unacceptable outcomes. As the moment of decision approached, each one of them basically collapsed and died with no other apparent cause. The crisis was an extreme failure of homeostasis, with parasympathetic dorsal-vagal-initiated freeze and cardiac arrest. When there is a sense of helplessness or stuckness in a situation, it can lead to death – perhaps this is the autoimmune issue. Where are you stuck? Where do you feel helpless? What are you struggling to make a decision about? Where in life does it not seem there is a positive way out? That recurrent worry about a financial problem or relationship conflict, that worry you seem to go over compulsively in your mind, contains many of the elements that cause the freeze response and many of the features of the classic approach/avoidance conflict: they are usually associated with things that you really desire (approach), but that also have a conflicting downside (avoidance). These negative and positive features create the state of helplessness that triggers the freeze response. I suggest that when you're in that state of detachment, filled with obsessive thinking about the conflict, you are in a state of dissociation, or the relative physiology of the freeze response. This is often exacerbated by a childhood adaptive coping mechanism of emotional self-suppression, significantly disabling the immune system.

In complex and repeated trauma, a person's environment may literally be packed with stimuli related in some way to old traumatic experiences. The images, emotions and somatic sensations can all be provoked, but without explicit memory, they cannot be articulated or understood. It's no wonder that trauma victims often suffer from agoraphobia – the fear of spaces, crowds, or any environment with many stimuli. These stimuli often trigger not only panic attacks but also many somatic complaints. Some somatic complaints, particularly pain, stiffness and muscle problems, are also related to triggers from environmental cues. The pathological alteration in the person's physiology is perfectly real. The perception of threat alters a sensitised person's brain and creates a visceral, physical symptom via the unstable ANS. Because of the sensitised wiring of circuits in the brain, people who have experienced life trauma are easily sensitised to virtually any sensory input. They respond to this input as a threat, which may result in hypervigilance and an exaggerated startle response, or perhaps spacing out and fogginess. This constant triggering is itself a stressor and a trauma. This sensitivity is quite common in the personalities of those with autoimmune conditions – it is perhaps the first thing I notice in the psychotherapy space.

So, trauma is characterised by the disruption of homeostasis. It affects both the brain and the essential systems of the body. The relative health of the brain depends on the health of the body, and vice versa. If trauma has adversely affected either one, you've got to find a means of healing that incorporates both brain and body: you can't fix one without fixing the other. The good news is that effective body-based psychotherapy can not only improve and correct the symptoms, but also promote the physical healing of damage to brain regions.

Attachment and early-life regulation as the foundation of the ANS

When children are born, their nervous systems have not yet fully developed. From birth to eighteen months, the nervous system is primarily moulded by the attachment to and interactions with the mother. The child-parent bond in the first two years is essential to the development of right brain structures responsible for autonomic, involuntary stress regulation and emotional regulation.

Like other mammals, humans are predisposed from birth to seek attachment to a caregiver for both safety and nurturing as well as a safe foundation from which to explore the outside world. If an infant is unable to form this primary attachment relationship with a caregiver, the infant adapts to the deficient caregiver by creating secondary attachment strategies. These attachment strategies have been classified as avoidant, anxious and disorganised. Working through childhood traumas and healing our early attachment styles through an integration of the mind and body is the key to restoring our intrinsic core intactness as well as to creating and sustaining healthy, meaningful adult relationships.

Secure attachment thrives when the holding environment is

safe and engenders basic trust. Parents are present and consistent, and show interest in and align with the child's state of mind. Communication is predictable, sensitive and attuned. Securely attached adults show realistic optimism in their world view, have a capacity for attunement and clear communication, and have resilience in recovering from stress, especially in relationships. These people tend to be unflappable and level-headed, and give others the benefit of the doubt when appropriate. They also demonstrate the capacity to initiate and receive repair attempts. For autoimmune conditions, people with secure attachments likely have the best protection – their nervous systems are capable of internal regulation, and a lack of trauma in the early years creates a hardy system. Chances are that those with a secure attachment may not develop autoimmune conditions at all due to their stable early environments.

Avoidant people tend to be relatively disconnected or dissociated from their physiology and/or their emotions. Avoidant attachment is usually the result of parents who were emotionally distant, rejecting and aversive to the child's signals of distress and bids for proximity. The child did not receive the mirroring or the exchange optimal for the development of the prefrontal cortex around emotional connectedness. Even memories and perceptions of the past are biologically detached in avoidant people – there needs to be an emotional connection for our brains to configure a personal memory, and a limbic connection for a 'feeling' memory to imprint. Avoidantly attached people describe their history in the same way as they approach relationships: the narrative is detached and impersonal. As an adult, one of such people's primary characteristics is being reliant solely on themselves, but unfortunately this is a self-reliance based on deficiency. It is an autonomy that is driven by fear and self-deprivation – an unhealthy, fear-driven autonomy. Due to the chronic bottling of emotions evident in the avoidant attachment style, it is likely that physical illness will manifest. The psychological issue gets stuck in the tissue of the body. This type could be said to feel too little.

In the anxious attachment style, children appear not to trust the consistent availability of the parent, always remaining overdependent, hypervigilant and hyperactivated in expression of needs. The child simultaneously feels hunger for closeness and a debilitating fear of losing the closeness. Anxious adults may experience chronic anxiety, frustration and despair in relationships, always expecting the worst of their partners. They have difficulty trusting themselves, their partners and their relationships. They will accept what they are given instead of asking clearly for what they want. They may 'give in order to get' and wonder why their partners sometimes feel angry instead of appreciative. Anxiously attached people feel that they must please their partners all the time to keep them. Often, there is a difficulty with the balance between giving and receiving. Due to chronic feelings of unsafeness, fear, worry and indecisiveness experienced by this attachment style, we can expect chronic ANS dysregulation. As the emotional triggers flood such people, their systems experience waves of adrenalin. This type could be said to feel too much. Burnout and chronic fatigue are common here.

In the disorganised attachment style, the infant displays chaotic and disoriented behaviour. The innate need to attach and the instinctual drive to survive are two major biological motivations that are constantly in conflict with one another. These people are equally terrified of intimacy and abandonment. Avoidance is motivated by a combination of the desperate need to connect with others so that they do not feel alone and have a safe haven in another, and the fear of being attacked. The main problem here is that two very strong psychobiological instinctive drives are in direct conflict – the need to attach and the need to survive danger. These children learn to suppress their self-protective instincts because their existence depends on frequently entering a harmful environment, which ultimately prevents them from being able to discern between safe and unsafe situations because their self-protective alarms no longer function. As adults, they may frequently dissociate and be attracted to danger, or be unaware that they are walking straight into it. They may not find options that are available to increase their safety. For example, abuse survivors often ignore the early signals of inappropriate behaviour from others, such as off-colour jokes, invasive touch and 'bad vibes'.

To heal, they may need to help bring these original survival instincts back into awareness and 'reactivate' this early-warning system. The therapist's goal is to bring the person with a disorganised attachment style out of dissociation and back into embodiment. There are often alternating patterns of flooding and dissociation that therapists want to lessen by helping these people to re-regulate the overarousal in their ANS. This chaotic state of feeling results in a constant adrenal state. This attachment style is most likely to develop autoimmune conditions. They could be said to experience misplaced feeling, as they are often living the triggers of the past as their present.

Healing attachment trauma is key to autoimmune conditions – this kind of trauma is the foundation of the dysregulation and is there before any symptoms begin. When I am doing psychotherapy, I imagine the adult as a child and what it was like for them from a very early age to begin to understand who they are now. People who have experienced attachment trauma frequently have hyperaroused bodies. The sympathetic nervous system is still active since it hasn't had an opportunity to discharge the trauma. After prolonged periods, the body–mind interprets the hyperaroused nervous system as normal. The threat response becomes internalised: the person no longer needs a tiger, an oncoming car, or a fire to trigger it. The threat response is brought on by the nervous system's own stored arousal. When this has been in the background throughout your life, your immune system does not stand a chance. The more disrupted your attachment period was, the less likely you'll have developed a solid base of resilience from which to operate, and the more likely you are to be overwhelmed by even small events later in your life – which then cause even greater dysregulation in your system.

Developmental trauma

We've seen that trauma causes biochemical alterations in the developing brain. Early adverse experiences have also been shown to initiate long-term changes in neurobiology, which may further increase vulnerability to psychological disturbances following subsequent stress. According to the stress-sensitisation hypothesis that early exposure to adversity alters the sensitivity of stress-response systems, like the HPA axis, which in turn enhances the risk of negative outcomes, including post-traumatic stress disorder

(PTSD), following later stressors. Findings of a growing number of studies indicate that the impact of trauma exposure may depend on the individual's age at the time of the event.

However, discrepant findings have emerged about the developmental period that most increases people's vulnerability to negative post-traumatic outcomes. There is evidence that traumatic events encountered during adolescence may be more central to one's identity, for example. When healing from trauma, we need to look at everything that has happened in life. We need to work through the core events and the domino effects of those events. Traumatic experiences create triggers. If, for example, you were once shouted at by a teacher, all teachers, including your second-year university lecturer, could elicit an anxious response from you. You may not even notice this response any more as it has been there for so long that you have become accustomed to it. The same applies to a car accident you had in your teens. There may now be a sub-noticeable fear every time you get into a car. What looks like a constant anxiety could be regular bouts of activation through subconscious memories being lifted into the now by present experience. Every person I have worked with who has an autoimmune presentation is experiencing multiple triggers within a day, and sometimes multiple triggers within each moment. The nervous system is on constant alert.

Research linking trauma to disease is still a developing field, although once you see this link it cannot be unseen. An adverse childhood experiences (ACE) study has documented the link between emotional trauma in childhood and physical difficulties in the body. This study found there to be predictive power between the two, in that an individual's number of ACEs predicted the amount of medical care required as an adult, with surprising accuracy. Individuals who had faced four or more categories of ACE were more likely to be diagnosed with cancer or autoimmune conditions than individuals who hadn't experienced childhood adversity. Someone with an ACE score of 4 was 460 per cent more likely to suffer from depression than someone with an ACE score of 0. An ACE score greater than or equal to 6 shortened an individual's lifespan by almost 20 years. Chronic central nervous system and body inflammation was found in these individuals. It's been discovered that chronic emotional stresses result in changes in gene functions (epigenetics) that enhance the risk of physical illness across a broad spectrum of conditions and augmented responses to stressors, leading to lives filled with chronic fear, anxiety and even severe psychiatric disorder. What were your prominent ACEs? How many of these experiences have you had? It is important to consider the traumas that did happen in your life – and, perhaps, the things that should have happened but never did.

Developmental trauma creates the narrative from which we lead our lives – the glasses we wear that may be tinted grey, and that colour our outlook on the world. Wouldn't it be nice to take those grey glasses off and put some rose-tinted ones on?

Trauma later in life

Trauma in the later years, such as relational trauma, can often bring autoimmunity to the fore. You've seen that relational trauma is trauma that happens in relationships. Often, we attract friends and lovers who form relationships that resemble the ones we had with our parents in some way. We re-enact past experiences through these relationships in an unconscious way, to attempt to resolve those experiences. In essence, the relationships we are in now reflect the level to which we have worked through our trauma. Many autoimmune conditions are triggered by characters who appear later in life and trigger repressed material from the relationships in our early years.

The psychological impact of trauma

Trauma has many psychological effects, but a few do stand out, and you can start looking at these. How our childhood trauma has caused us to conduct ourselves may open us up to being taken advantage of, abused, overworked, overextended and other features that are common in the typical autoimmune personality. These psychological effects of trauma become causal and maintaining factors for autoimmune conditions in themselves. They include our boundaries, how positively or negatively we define ourselves (our beliefs and self-love), our assertiveness (our power to stand up for ourselves), our ability to live spontaneously in a childlike, creative manner (in a state of flow), and the way we engage with the world around us (our personality or identity). When working psychotherapeutically with those with autoimmune conditions, boundaries, assertiveness and authenticity are important areas – and working on them often uncovers deeply buried childhood traumas.

Boundaries mean knowing your limits and not letting others infringe on them. They allow us to coexist with others who have different ideas and ways of life. We learn boundaries in our developmental trauma and our early interactions. We can have porous, rigid or healthy boundaries. Porous boundaries are things such as oversharing information, lack of communication about boundaries, difficulty saying no, accepting disrespect or abuse, and overinvolvement in others' problems. Porous boundaries take the form of enmeshed relationships, people-pleasing and saving others. Developmentally, you may have been in an enmeshed relationship with one of your parents (where they overshared their emotional difficulties with you), or in a highly dependent relationship. This difficult relationship often continues into adulthood, making it very hard to untie the relationship between the two people so that each person is their own individual. So, the adult child either has difficulty finding themselves in a relationship of their own, or forms co-dependent relationships.

People-pleasing is another presentation of porous boundaries, often having its roots in pacifying a difficult parent. It happens when you have a difficult time saying no to others. It indicates that you depend on others for approval because your sense of value comes from outside yourself instead of within yourself. You fear rejection, so you do whatever it takes to avoid it: this was a survival strategy for you as a child. As children we cannot be rejected, as our survival depends on being connected to our caregivers. If we are raised in environments where there is conditional acceptance based on our achieving or behaving in a particular manner, we learn not to love and value ourselves as we are, and we ensure that we fit in with the ideals that are set up for us. We then strive constantly to be who we need to be to be accepted. This, in my opinion, is the psychological source of burnout (and chronic fatigue) – pushing ourselves beyond our own limits, not being who we truly are, and always searching for that external approval we never fully managed to obtain from our parental figures.

Trying to save others is another form of porous boundaries in action. This is when we make another person our focus, often at our own expense, and try save them from their difficulties. If we had a depressed or anxious parent, it may have been the norm to try to cheer them up – this is also a way to survive, as a depressed parent will not take care of you effectively, so it is in your best interests to cheer them up. We can see that all these patterns of relating to our caregivers in our early years determine how we relate to others in terms of boundaries in our later relationships.

Advice for those with porous boundaries: focus on yourself. Those with porous boundaries can be likened to those with an anxious attachment style. Porous boundaries are a defining feature of the autoimmune personality.

On the opposite end of the spectrum, we get rigid boundaries. This looks like: being detached, keeping others at a distance, avoiding intimacy, difficulty asking for help, and being overly private or protective about personal information. Those with rigid boundaries often appear coldhearted. The healthy vulnerability and empathy of a fulfilling relationship is often substituted with indifference, callousness and apathy. Those with rigid boundaries can be found being quite intolerant of others and have high expectations of them.

Rigidity is also found in people who cannot take constructive criticism, typically because they are sensitive and fear feeling rejected. You will often find that these individuals are made of brick – they are fixed and stubborn, and cannot be shifted. This is how they have learnt to cope with the unpredictability of their childhood. The more in control and unchangeable they are in the present, the more they can control the present's unpredictability. Often, this kind of person does not do well in spontaneous environments (travelling to African countries, for example) or where others need to take the lead (being a passenger in a plane).

People with rigid boundaries are less likely to share the challenges they are facing or intimate parts of their lives with you as they may not have experienced growing up in an environment where someone truly cared about hearing this information. Sharing this kind of information may also have been detrimental, leading to punishment. Many men have been raised in such a way, with emotional expression being punished. Rigid individuals live in a form of isolation in that they have superficial or guarded relationships with others, avoiding close connection.

Advice for those with rigid boundaries: *surrender and open up*. Those with rigid boundaries can be likened to those with an avoidant attachment style. Rigid boundaries are common in some autoimmune manifestations, such as rheumatoid arthritis.

Finally, healthy boundaries – this looks like not compromising your values, sharing in an appropriate or balanced way, knowing and communicating your needs, and respecting others' thoughts and desires. If you are able to say no when you feel uncomfortable with a situation, you are setting healthy boundaries. If you take time to listen to your own needs and opinions when you make decisions, you are much less likely to find yourself in a compromised position. When you have healthy boundaries, you come across as caring and compassionate, without being overly emotional. Others realise that you are someone they can turn to for support when they need it – but in this position you don't feel overextended, and you don't seek validation from supporting others.

Boundaries and our personality (or coping personality) have a strong link. Our personality develops through all the interactions we have at a young age (with a prominent focus on the traumas we experience). I have had some patients who became everything their parents wanted or needed them to be in their early years. People become who they needed while they were experiencing the traumas of their lives. This makes them miss out on who they truly are. It is likely that you project your unmet childhood need onto others in this way – being their fixer as no one took you to the doctor when you were young, being their rescuer as you had to endure years of your parents fighting. Shifting out of our coping personality into our true, authentic self involves working through the traumas that created the coping parts and releasing the emotion that holds us to that way of being. It needs us to recognise our coping personality and the fact that it is fuelled by deficient boundaries.

A pleaser coping personality is chameleon-like, shapeshifting into whatever is suited to the present situation. This malleability develops as a response to caregivers who require agreeableness to respond favourably to the child. If children in this situation assert their true selves, they would likely be subjected to abuse, and they often lose their identity somewhere along the way. The pleaser personality requires self-silencing, which is where suppression of your own emotions is born. Often, in this action, a great deal of anger is buried. Healing the pleaser in psychotherapy often means accessing a mountain of anger suppressed over the lifetime. People with the nurturer or carer coping personality may have had a caregiver who suffered from depression or a physical illness. They now nurture and care for others, projecting the missing parts of their experience onto others. These personalities often compulsively do for and help others, and not themselves. People with an achiever or performer coping personality (often presenting as a Type A personality and very prone to burnout) sought the validation of a caregiver as children. Perhaps they feel that they were never able to reach their caregivers' ideals. These people rarely celebrate and hold feelings of accomplishment for very long, often moving from accomplishment to accomplishment in a never-ending search for the illusive approval of the original caregiver. Often, all these specific traits can be traced back to exact trauma events.

People with the coping personalities I've explained all expend a lot of effort in maintaining these personalities and are prone to burnout. The combination of these personalities is what I call the autoimmune personality. Ayurvedic practitioners have also established an autoimmune coping personality, according to which autoimmunity is more frequently exhibited in those who are deeply ethically or morally conflicted and highly idealistic. When your actions don't line up with your internal moral standard, you become stressed and despondent. They are often critical of themselves and prone to low self-esteem. To heal, they may need to relax this 'moral code' and be more practical about life, which may mean less 'I must/I need to/I should' and more of just letting the river of life take you where it wants you to go. A list of the names I have identified from among my autoimmune patients for their coping personalities includes: pleaser, achiever, performer, perfectionist, outsider, fixer, black sheep, manager, the responsible one, survivor, victim, the bad one, and the controlling one. This list is by no means all-encompassing and perhaps you can identify a few more. The survival roles you acquired in childhood helped you with the adversity and pain of that time and coalesced to form who you are. Your autoimmune diagnosis is now telling you those roles are no longer appropriate and that it is time to create a new way of being in the world.

Research is showing us that outgoing, sociable people have the strongest immune systems. Extraverts are often gregarious and conversational, and tend to take the lead and seek out new experiences. Extraverts typically have stronger social abilities, experience more pleasant emotions and have higher levels of motivation. Those who are the most conscientious and careful, though, are most likely to have a weaker immune system response. Conscientious people are systematic and dutiful, more likely to follow through on their plans than their less conscientious peers. This is typical in the Type A personality.

Assertiveness, or standing up for yourself, is the access point to shifting your boundaries and coping personality. This involves activating the disciplined, focused, non-negotiating, firm, take-no-shit part of yourself. This part may need some practice to come into action. Having spent so much time in a passive, passive-aggressive, *walking-on-eggshells*, or even aggressive state may result in some awkwardness in finding your true voice. When this voice initially comes out it may be unsure or shaky, and it may elicit shame and guilt. This shame and guilt are those childhood emotions you experienced if this voice came out back then. Feel those feelings, then roar louder. As you experience your assertiveness without those childhood consequences – and perhaps even some external validation – your voice will become more certain. Healing will require you to own all the aspects of yourself by being brave and courageous, and able to go outside the norm and be fully yourself. You will need to let go of the parts of yourself that are seeking approval, or of gatekeeping all those things you could potentially lose.

When your inner child comes into contact with something that shifts its frequency out of the tone of play, joy and flow, the assertive part of you can immediately act to protect the child's frequency, so that the child can resume what it needs to resume. You will need to develop the subtlety of identifying the things that shift the child's frequency through listening to your inner core. This is part of developing your assertiveness – being true to what is best for you and not veering from that.

 Task

Many people who have autoimmune conditions have been walking on eggshells with others all their lives. Put this book down right now and find a mirror. Look into your own eyes and roar as loudly as you possibly can. Practise this daily until the discomfort of doing it is gone.

Assertiveness is linked to various beliefs: if I speak up, there will be consequences; if I say no, I will be in trouble; good girls are agreeable and don't speak unless spoken to. What memories are linked to your beliefs about being assertive? Was there anyone who was assertive in your family home? Please discriminate here between 'assertive' and 'aggressive'. An assertive response creates a space where others are able to respond assertively. Psychological assertiveness creates internal boundaries that manifest in physical boundaries inside the body – for example, a stronger gut lining and a stronger nervous system.

Negative beliefs have their origins in trauma

As we grow up, and especially as we experience trauma, we acquire various beliefs about ourselves and others: I am not good enough; I am not safe; I am not lovable; I am bad; I am alone; men are dangerous; women are weak; and so forth. The beliefs 'I am not safe' and 'I am alone' frequently come up when I am working with people who have autoimmune conditions. Another common belief is 'I must caretake today, so that I am taken care of tomorrow'. We project these beliefs onto the world, and in this way we co-create the experience of this being affirmed.

Imagine that inside you was a beautiful, wise fairy godmother. Each time one of these negative beliefs came up, she would invalidate it, root you to where its origins are in your memory, express to you that you were only an innocent child when that took place and that is not your fault, and finally replace that negative belief with one that will better serve you in life and be more aligned with the truth of the perfection of your being. Self-love may seem like an 'airy fairy godmother' concept, but this is the core of what you need to activate in your life. When you engage in life from a positive set of self-beliefs, you set yourself up for positive patterns and experience – you manifest what you truly want. What are your core negative beliefs? How are they affecting your life? With which more useful things can you replace them?

Your patterns, the way your parents took care of you (or didn't take care of you), the way you saw your parents take care of themselves and each other – these form your patterns of self-care. People with autoimmune conditions often have patterns of neglect, abuse, self-sacrifice, or something similar in their history. Look deeply at how you look after yourself, how kind you are to yourself, how much you allow yourself to receive from others, how much fun you allow yourself to have, how much time you allow for connection versus work, how much suffering you allow, or how readily you shift yourself into more pleasant places and states. Deep inside, your inner child believes, 'I deserve this'. Make sure your inner child gets something special from this life – a joyous adventure, love, play, being cared for, being someone's best thing, and work that involves creative expression. Which patterns have you noticed keep repeating in your life? What keeps happening, over and over? What keeps happening in your romantic relationships? Is this similar to the experience you had with your parents in childhood? Could there be something you keep doing over and over to elicit the repeating of these things?

Each traumatic experience has the capacity to take us back a few hundred steps – or to be a path to transformation and the development of even greater resilience in the face of future blows. You are your greatest parenting tool. None of us was perfectly parented. We all have wounds of the heart that we picked up on our journey to adulthood. We all need to embark on a journey of healing and restoration. The ancient shamanic cultures call trauma 'soul loss', which can be likened to a loss of life force. Boundaries and energetic frequency are important words here in getting this life force back.

If this section has left you with a feeling of discomfort, please contact a psychotherapist. You may need to work through this. Reading about trauma can be very triggering.

Adrenaline

Adrenaline is the hormone of stress and trauma, so it is a good next port of call. Also called epinephrine, it is a hormone released by your adrenal glands and some neurons. The adrenal glands are located at the top of each kidney. They are responsible for producing many hormones, including aldosterone, cortisol, adrenaline and noradrenaline. The adrenal glands are controlled by another gland called the pituitary gland. The adrenal glands are divided into two parts: outer glands (adrenal cortex) and inner glands (adrenal medulla). The inner glands produce adrenaline.

Adrenaline is also known as the fight-or-flight hormone. It's released in response to stressful, exciting, dangerous and threatening situations. Adrenaline helps your body react quickly. It makes the heart beat faster, increases blood flow to the brain and muscles, and stimulates the body to make sugar to use for fuel. Once in the bloodstream, adrenaline:

- binds to receptors on liver cells to break down larger sugar molecules, called glycogen, into a smaller, more readily usable form called glucose; this gives your muscles a boost of energy
- binds to receptors on muscle cells in the lungs, causing you to breathe faster
- stimulates cells of the heart to beat faster
- triggers the blood vessels to contract and direct blood towards the major muscle groups
- contracts muscle cells below the surface of the skin to stimulate perspiration
- binds to receptors on the pancreas to inhibit the production of insulin.

As you can see, it has a huge and extensive impact on the various systems of your body. I can't help making the link between diabetes and adrenaline here, as in the first point above. Adrenaline is certainly linked to most other illnesses in a complex interaction with the immune system. While the fight-or-flight response is very useful when it comes to avoiding a car accident or running away from a lion, it can be a problem when it's activated in response to everyday stress. Your body is stimulated to release adrenaline and other stress-related hormones, such as cortisol (commonly known as the stress hormone), when your mind is filled with thoughts, anxiety and concern. This is especially true at night when you're lying in bed in a calm, dark, unstimulated atmosphere and all of a sudden you find yourself fixated on a fight from the previous day or wondering about what will happen tomorrow. While your brain perceives this as stress, real danger isn't actually present. This can leave you feeling restless and irritable and make it impossible to fall asleep.

We have long lived in a toxic, work-hard-play-hard culture in most of the western world that is presenting with ever-increasing autoimmunity and other stress-related conditions. If we go up the river to find out why people are falling into this adrenaline pattern, we can see that much of society functions in this way. We have created a world in which we are always reaching for something more. We are stuck in a perpetual cycle of overwork and depletion. Advertising and media of various kinds push us to this place through promoting materialism. We see what we want, and we work harder to get it. Not many manage to escape this perpetual seeking.

Adrenaline allows us to escape from danger in that it shuts us off from various parts of ourselves – like our ability to feel pain. Adrenaline has the same effect on our body whether a real threat is present or not. Our ability to feel pain is rather important – pain signals to us that something is not right inside. It draws our attention to the problem so that we can resolve it. When we are living in a chronic adrenal state (driven by stress and trauma), this signal has been switched off. The signal of our health and well-being has been turned down.

In essence, living on adrenaline disconnects us from ourselves. We work all week in a highly adrenal state and then arrive at the weekend when, to release our stress, we use various substances – the main one being alcohol – or extreme coping behaviour, such as cycling 100 kilometres. It is important for us to know that, when our bodies are running on adrenaline, they are not restoring themselves. Fight-or-flight mode shuts down the functions in the body that are not required for immediate survival, like digestion and cell regeneration. The fight-or-flight response is all about immediate survival, often at the expense of long-term health. If adrenaline is on, the immune system is turned down; digestion and thus nutrient absorption is turned down; and we are in survival mode. There is no rest, and without rest there cannot be restoration.

Adrenaline is the foundation of autoimmunity. During the fight, flight or freeze response, the brain releases a large volume of endorphins – the brain's pain-suppressing chemicals. For example, soldiers in battle have been documented to have increased pain tolerance for hours after their injuries. This is a survival mechanism that helps us continue, to enhance our chances of survival despite the pain. This very mechanism is how we break our bodies and move into autoimmunity. Our disconnection from our bodies, as well as a flood of reinforcing adrenaline and endorphins for extended periods, means we can't feel the exhaustion, the pain and the damage happening within.

Adrenaline may also be released as a response to loud noises, bright lights and high temperatures – stressors in our environment. Watching television, using your smartphone or computer, or listening to loud music before bedtime can contribute to a surge of adrenaline at night. I believe that smartphones are playing quite a big role in the increase in autoimmune and related diagnoses. Research suggests that phone-induced anxiety operates on a positive feedback loop: our phones keep us in a persistent state of anxiety, and the only relief from this anxiety is to look at our phones. According to this same research, most people experience an emotional response that floods their body with stress hormones when they hear their phone go off. Physiological arousal spikes quite a bit after each text comes in.

Other recent studies suggest that, on average, Americans unlock their phones approximately 100 times a day. Whether you're checking the time, sending a text or googling a fact, each interaction can cause stress. When you check your phone or hear an alert, you activate your sympathetic nervous system, the part of your body that's always scanning the environment. It gives you a little shot of adrenaline for every interaction. That adrenaline, which is meant to trigger your body to pay attention, sets off a cascade of chemicals that increase heart rate, pulse and muscle tension, and redirects energy from the brain to the muscles. It takes 5 to 30 minutes for your body to get back to its baseline after every one of these alarms.

It leaves me wondering whether we ever come back to our baselines.

All this stress wreaks havoc on the body and mind, causing or contributing to a range of diseases, from heart disease and depression to sleep deprivation and chronic fatigue. This is strongly at play as a causal factor in autoimmune activation. Platforms like Facebook, Snapchat and Instagram leverage the very same neural circuitry used by slot machines and cocaine to keep us using their products as much as possible. Dopamine is a chemical produced by our brains that plays a starring role in motivating behaviour. It gets released when we take a bite of delicious food, when we have sex, after we exercise, and, importantly, when we have successful social interactions. In an evolutionary context, it rewards us for beneficial behaviours and motivates us to repeat them. Although not as intense as hit of cocaine, positive social stimuli similarly result in a release of dopamine, reinforcing whatever behaviour preceded it. The same dopaminergic reward circuits are activated by gratifying social cues like laughing faces, positive peer acknowledgment and communications from loved ones, according to cognitive neuroscientists. Smartphones have provided us with a virtually unlimited supply of social stimuli, both positive and negative. Every notification, whether it's a text message, a like on Instagram, or a Facebook notification, has the potential to be a dopamine-inducing social stimulus. In addition, the blue light from smartphone and computer screens stimulates the adrenal system and dysregulates the neurotransmitter balance in the brain. If you wake up in the morning and immediately seek your phone, you are surging your body with adrenaline from the very start. Perhaps yoga or a swim would be a better way to start your day.

Ask yourself these questions:

- Why are you using your phone like this?
- What do you gain from this experience? Is this a valid or real gain?
- Are you lonely and disconnected from others?
- Does your life not have enough joy in it?
- Is it that you want to show the world who you are, or attract someone?
- What are you searching for in your phone that you are not finding in your life? You need to address that.

High temperatures stimulate an adrenal response. According to TCM, high temperatures fire up your yang. Excess yang looks like aggression, irritability and difficulties with concentration. The place where you are living may be firing up your adrenals in terms of daily temperature. I recommend keeping yourself warm and comfortable, with no extremes, while you are healing.

It is worth considering the activities you engage in from an adrenaline perspective. If you are spending your weekends parachuting out of planes with a developing autoimmune disease, it could be time to rethink your hobbies until your system can cope with them. Often, people with a history of childhood trauma are prone to not feeling much in the ordinary moments of joy, often chasing more extreme stimulation to relieve their boredom and feel more than mundane, ordinary life. The nervous system may need to become accustomed to the ordinary in life again and let go of the stimulation-seeking that has been patterned as a way of maintaining the adrenal activation of childhood.

Something that is even more vital to look at is what kind of adrenaline you experience at work. This is often a bit harder to change, but change is needed nonetheless. A high-voltage work environment might be keeping you on your toes in a way that is eating up your immune resilience.

Another area to look at is the people you engage with – how calm or chaotic they are. If you are surrounded by emotionally dysregulated, unpredictable or aggressive people, it may be time to rethink your circles. If you had a difficult childhood and are living with your family of origin, it may mean you are regularly triggered. The adrenal spike every time you face a trigger may mean a constant flow of adrenaline through the system. Your home needs to be a space that feels like a sanctuary. Where you live needs to be physically safe and serene, not only in terms of the people in the environment. Do you feel safe in your own home, community, body and mind? Is this illness playing a protective role in your life? Sometimes it serves one to stay in the illness as a means of receiving the care and support that was previously absent, pacifying conflict in your home environment, avoiding a toxic career, or keeping yourself at home, reducing exposure to stress and trauma. In these ways, and others, your illness may come to serve a function and your unconscious may work to maintain it to protect you.

Consider, too, the type of content you watch on TV and when you watch TV. It can be a good wind-down, but it also feeds your system with material that is imprinted into you. Many use TV as a relief from boredom, living through the characters they get exposed to. I am very careful about the content I consume as I have recognised that this becomes you – how you think and what you project onto your life. Picture what happens in your body when you watch a horror movie or a thriller – what you are emotionally putting yourself through, and what your adrenals are doing. Does your psyche discriminate between this being reality or fiction? I have many patients who compulsively watch the news and have seen the dysregulation this has brought. If you are going to watch something, let it be valuable in some way to you – or at least offer you some fantasy escape that leaves you feeling comforted and relaxed, rather than hypervigilant. Disney movies and their music are often the right recipe for relaxing parasympathetic activation and bringing you into a regulated state.

Polyvagal theory

Perhaps this is a good time to take a detour and explain Stephen Porges's polyvagal theory. According to this theory, there are three strategies the body may use when experiencing a threat: immobility, fight or flight, or social engagement.

When a person is immobile, they collapse, their muscles become limp, and they enter a condition of altered consciousness and complete exhaustion. To escape being attacked by its alleged predator, the body essentially pretends to be dead. This is sometimes referred to as the freeze-or-fawn response. The fight-or-flight response is what most of us are more familiar with. Humans are naturally inclined to look for pleasure and to steer clear of discomfort. When a threat is close by, we feel motivated to flee, and the body responds by getting us ready to either leave or attack. When external factors or our bodies fail to defend us by following the right biological defence protocol in the face of an overwhelming threat, the energy that has been activated cannot be released effectively, which results in traumatisation. This fight-or-flight neural energy brain subsystem evolved from the reptilian period nearly 300 million years ago and is the domain of the reptilian brain.

Social engagement is the third and most recently acquired tactic. Humans are social creatures who depend, and are interdependent, on the relationships they build with others. People will presumably try to safeguard those relationships and thereby themselves. This is why, when someone is angry with us, we try to defend or explain ourselves verbally so that the person will not lash out at us. If, like animals, we do not immediately fight or flee, the energy becomes stuck in our nervous system, requiring release in some form later. We are intellectual beings, and our intellect and intelligence have developed in accordance with the functions of our physical bodies. So, when we are feeling stressed or threatened by a person or a relationship, we do not usually want to attack that person physically or run away. But we may want to protect ourselves by protecting the relationship itself, or by releasing our pent-up survival energy in a verbal manner, which would require us to talk things out with family, friends, or the ones who are close to us. A malfunction in this third strategy, social engagement, is often closely related to a person's attachment issues and trauma.

The ANS is the master regulator of the endocrine and gut functions that sustain stability and homeostasis. It specifically works on the fight-or-flight sympathetic nervous system (excitation), and the vegetative, rest/restore parasympathetic nervous system (relaxation). Each state – fight or flight/freeze or fawn, exertion/rest, seeking/ digesting food, sympathetic/parasympathetic – involves opposites. Staying in one of these states for too long negatively affects the body, causing significant distress and disease. Yet both opposites are essential for survival.

The vagus nerve is the nerve concerned with the fight-or-flight response. What is important for you to know is that it is linked to many important parts of the body, so we can say that it has an influence on many systems. If we look at all the organs it innervates, the link between the various autoimmune symptoms and adrenaline becomes clear. The vagus nerve even inputs into the ear, and here we see symptoms like tinnitus presenting.

The smooth muscles of the stomach and intestines are strongly affected by the dorsal aspect of the vagus nerve, which largely innervates the sub-diaphragm (although it also has some connections to the heart and lungs). This neural system controls digestion and urination in addition to regulating freeze and death-feigning behaviours when a threat to life is present. The upper thoracic structures, including the heart and lungs, are largely innervated by the ventral aspect of the vagus nerve. The vagus nerve and other cranial nerves can communicate in both directions. The neural circuits that regulate the utilization of the muscle groups used in social interaction behaviours are specifically implicated. This includes the nerves that control the larynx and pharynx (used for producing speech used in verbal communication), the muscles in the middle ear (used for tuning the eardrum to extract the speech of others from our complex acoustic environment), and facial muscles (used for expression and engagement), as well as others. These nerves are the infrastructure used by social mammals to engage with other individuals, and the activation of this complex appears to be a primary pathway for the parasympathetic system to calm human physiology. Safe connection pacifies our fight-or-flight response.

According to psychotherapist Peter Levine, when your nervous system becomes overwhelmed and threatened by an unexpected, unwanted stimulus, the body innately and automatically takes certain sequential biological steps, as the organism goes into survival mode, to regulate the nervous system and rebalance the body. The ANS is responsible for this self-regulation, acting as a control system and prompting the body to return to normalcy. If a threat is perceived, the individual engages in self-protective responses modulated by the different branches of the ANS.

As you've seen, the difference between how humans and animals experience threats lies in humans' use of the left brain. When the social engagement system is dominant, the individual may try to consciously assess the situation, call out for help, or attempt other social strategies to defuse the threat. If these are unsuccessful, the sympathetic nervous system (SNS) is employed to support mobilisation behaviours, or active coping. When people feel threatened, a rapid cascade of non-conscious survival responses is generated. Sensory inputs are processed rapidly in the amygdala (the smoke detector of the brain), which mobilises a predictable threat response cycle when stimuli are tagged as dangerous. This is the fight-or-flight response. If these responses are unsuccessful, the freeze response will ensue, with collapse inducing quiescence. This biophysiological cascade follows an evolutionarily determined trajectory, in which the body relies on more recently evolved – and more adaptive – systems first.

If the organism successfully defuses a threat at any point in this process, the body is designed to downregulate, releasing the survival energy mobilised to manage dangerous situations. People may report waves of heat, which often shift to warmth as deactivation occurs. As the system settles, mild vibration, shaking or tingling sensations may be felt. The parasympathetic nervous system may cause the lachrymal glands to release tears, resulting in crying. In these and other ways, the body may enact its instinctual and intelligent response to highly stressing scenarios, releasing the accumulated overactivation and returning the organism to efficient equilibrium and homeostasis. It is when this does not occur that an organism is vulnerable to accumulated stress or traumatisation.

Window of tolerance

Psychiatry professor Dan Siegel's window of tolerance is a model to help us function more optimally. All of our emotions fluctuate, particularly at times of crisis and stress. The window of tolerance describes the best state of 'arousal' or stimulation in which we are able to function and thrive in everyday life. When we function within this window, we are able to learn effectively, play and relate well to others and ourselves. However, if we move outside of this window, we can become hyper- or hypo-aroused.

Hyperarousal results from the fight-or-flight response and is characterised by excessive energy or activation. It can present as difficulties concentrating, irritability, anger and angry outbursts, panic, constant anxiety, being easily scared or startled, and self-destructive behaviour. Hypo-arousal results from the freeze or the flop response, where there is a sense of shutting down or disassociating. This can present as exhaustion, depression, flat affect, numbness and disconnection.

We all have different 'windows' due to factors like our significant childhood experiences, neurobiology, social support, environment and coping skills. The size of our windows can change from day to day. The wider the window, the less likely we are to experience anger or frustration, or to feel flat and lack energy.

WINDOW OF TOLERANCE
The window of tolerance and the different states that affect you

HYPERAROUSAL
- Abnormal state of increased responsiveness
- Feeling anxious, angry and out of control
- You may experience wanting to fight or run away

DYSREGULATION
- When you start to deviate outside your window of tolerance you start to feel agitated, anxious, or angry
- You do not feel comfortable but you are not out of control yet

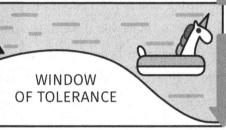

Think of the window of tolerance as a river and you're floating down it. When the river narrows, it's fast and unsafe. When it widens, it slows down and you:
- are at a balanced and calm state of mind
- feel relaxed and in control
- are able to function more effectively
- are able to take on any challenge life throws at you

Meditation, listening to music, or engaging hobbies can expand your window of tolerance

SHRINK
your Window of Tolerance

Stress and trauma can cause your window of tolerance to shrink

WINDOW OF TOLERANCE

EXPAND
your Window of Tolerance

DYSREGULATION
- You start to feel overwhelmed, your body might start shutting down and you could lose track of time
- You do not feel comfortable but you are not out of control yet

HYPERAROUSAL
- Abnormal state of decreased responsiveness
- Feeling emotional numbness, exhaustion, and depression
- You may experience your body shutting down or freeze

© Mind My Peelings

84

You can think of your window of tolerance as a river that you're floating down. When you expand your window of tolerance the river widens, and the flow slows down. You are comfortable and safe flowing with the calm waters, able to tolerate whatever life brings to you. However, when you experience adversity, trauma, undue stress or anxiety, your window of tolerance shrinks. The river begins to narrow and the flow of the water speeds up. You start to feel uncomfortable and unsafe, and have difficulty keeping yourself afloat. Small stressors overwhelm you. The window of tolerance thus determines your resilience.

If you have an autoimmune condition, it is likely that your window of tolerance is narrow, and that you have been long disconnected from the action of your adrenals. It's time to take cognisance of this and begin to notice where you are. Creating this internal awareness is called interoception. It means beginning to watch the fluctuations in your body from the inside out. It is likely that you have been stuck on 'on' for a very long time, which may be due to your trauma history. The best way to expand your window of tolerance is to expose yourself to stressors, only to a level that you can handle and gradually increasing this as your tolerance increases.

Task

Getting our adrenals under control is fundamental in healing autoimmune conditions. Make a list of all the things that cause your body to release adrenaline in your daily life. Take a fine-tooth comb and think about everything. Do you have a chaotic pet? What is the quality of the alarm that wakes you up in the morning? Consider each and every aspect of your day that you can start to address to lower your adrenal load.

Genetics

We are all born with certain Achilles heels, or weaker areas, in our body. There are typically inherited. If your mother has thyroid problems, it is possible that you may experience this. The key word here, however, is *possible*. We require environmental factors, such as stress, environmental toxins or the types of foods we eat, to activate these inherited predispositions. So, our lifestyle, behaviours and the things we are exposed to can alter the way our genes operate.

As Dan Siegel says, 'nature needs nurture'. You may never experience the health problems that run in your family if you have protective factors in the form of a healthy lifestyle (diet, exercise and low stress) and a positive life experience (good support and low levels of trauma experienced through your lifetime). Eating a diet low in fats, calories and salt may mitigate the expression of a genetic tendency for obesity, diabetes, coronary artery disease or hypertension. Your genes play an important role in your health, but so do your behaviours and environment. Epigenetics is the study of how your behaviours and environment can cause changes that affect the way your genes work – it is the science that studies when these genes are turned on and off. Unlike genetic changes, epigenetic changes are reversible and do not change your DNA sequence, but they can change how your body reads a DNA sequence.

In recent years, studies in genetic inheritance have begun to show that certain types of life experience seem to affect family members several generations down the line in mysterious and unexpected ways. These findings have cast considerable doubt on our assumptions about the inevitability of our genetic heritage. They suggest that other, previously unidentified, factors are at work here. This epigenetic inheritance means that health issues you are experiencing could have originated with the behaviour, diet and environment of your parents, grandparents and great-grandparents.

For generations, scientists have assumed that DNA, the genetic material that governs our genetic inheritance, is stable, unchangeable and inevitable, and that it determines the transmission of traits. But in the past decade or so, it has become apparent that external forces can 'switch on' or 'switch off' parts of our genetic code, a process called transcription. And once changed, that altered code can continue to be passed on for generations. This should be considered in post-traumatic generational trauma as well.

Research on the interactions between environmental and genetic factors aims to explain why autoimmunity afflicts certain individuals and not others. Epigenetic dysregulation directly influences the development of autoimmunity by regulating immune cell functions. The recognition of the complexity of the interaction between epigenetic events and the alteration of the immune system in autoimmune disorders is a prominent challenge for the discovery of novel potential therapeutic strategies. Particular life experiences in certain critical periods may inhibit or activate the copying of one or more genes that may ultimately result in health problems. Pathogens such as viruses can change your epigenetics to weaken your immune system. This helps those viruses to survive.

Perhaps epigenetics represents our biochemical or scientific basis of karma – patterns that get created over time. We live the karma of our past generations' actions through our minds and our bodies. Clearing that karma means coming to awareness of those old patterns and creating new ones to replace them. In recent years, I have become interested in learning more about my parents' lives and even the lives of my grandparents, as there is no doubt that our psychological makeup and even neuroses are directly related to their experiences.

Is there autoimmunity in your family? What side is it on? What traumas have been experienced in that family line? Did a particular event activate your autoimmunity? Is that event similar to what your family members with the condition experienced? Or is that a persistent pattern that repeats in your family in some way?

Bacteria, fungi, viruses and other infections

In essence, autoimmunity is the stuck regulation inherent in PTSD, causing a flood of adrenaline and chronic cortisol, which disables the immune system and activates or invites pathogens. The symptoms of PTSD procedural memory, coupled with the symptoms of the body under attack from a virus, form the symptoms of an autoimmune condition.

I can say with near certainty that there is some kind of parasite, bacterium, virus or fungus living inside you at present. You are being host to something and that something is parasitically feeding off you and often making you chronically fatigued. Possibly through stress or trauma, this pathogen has come to the fore and is manifesting in your present symptoms. Many of the patients presenting in my practice these days engage in psychiatry and psychotherapy with no symptom relief. On deeper investigation it is clear that anxiety, depression, ADHD and even bipolar diagnoses could be rooted in a viral, fungal or bacterial (or combined) infection.

Parasites are organisms that live off the host and get their food from or at the expense of the host. Parasites leach your nutrients from your body. Physical and psychological boundaries determine your susceptibility to parasites. Symptoms of parasites may include mood fluctuations, cravings for processed and sugary foods, iron deficiency, skin ailments, yeast infections, bleeding gums, headaches, anxiety, teeth grinding, food allergies, fatigue, digestive problems, brain fog and heart palpitations.

Most people out there seem to have a candida overgrowth in the gut. We all have candida to some degree; it is the overgrowth or imbalance that points to something difficult for the body (and this having a knock-on effect on the mind as candida has much to do with our moods). According to Louise Hay, candida is metaphysically (or psychologically) linked to feeling scattered, lots of frustration and anger, and demanding and untrusting relationships. People with candida often complain of ADHD-like symptoms – attention difficulties, a feeling of being disorganised and mentally clouded. Candida can be alleviated with probiotics and diet changes. Gluten, sugar (especially from alcohol) and dairy are big culprits in feeding candida.

Here is a partial list of infections that have been linked to autoimmunity, which I have seen in patients or that have been reported in research. Part of this list has been extracted from Izabella Wentz's *Hashimoto's Protocol*:

- *Bartonella henselae*, or cat scratch fever
- Bilharzia
- *Blastocystis hominis*
- *Borrelia burgdorferi*, the bacterium that causes Lyme disease
- *Brucella*

- *Candida albicans*
- *Chlamydia pneumoniae*
- *Chlamydia psitacci*
- *Chlamydia trachomatis*
- *Coxiella burnetii*
- Coxsackievirus
- *Cryptosporidium*
- Cytomegalovirus
- *Dientamoeba fragilis*
- Epstein-Barr virus (EBV)
- *Endolimax nana*
- *Entamoeba histolytica*
- Enterovirus
- Erythrovirus B19
- *Giardia lamblia*
- *Helicobacter pylori*
- Hepatitis C
- Herpes viruses
- Human parvovirus
- Human T-lymphotropic virus type 1 (HTLV-1)
- *Iodamoeba bütschlii*
- Mumps
- *Mycobacterium avium subspecies paratuberculosis*
- *Mycoplasma pneumoniae*
- Rickettsia
- Rubella
- Sinus infections
- Small intestinal bacterial overgrowth (SIBO)

- Streptococcal exo-enzymes
- *Toxoplasma gondii*
- *Yersinia enterocolitica.*

It is estimated that 97 per cent of people have EBV – the 'kissing disease'. It is so easy to catch this from forks at restaurants and even that stranger you passionately kissed on Saturday night – it's no wonder all this chronic illness is ever-increasing.

EBV infection is glandular fever. The virus resides in our livers and becomes activated through stress and trauma or co-infection such as COVID-19. Our immune systems change and may weaken as we become older, bringing any dormant viruses to the fore. You'll recall that Louise Hay believes EBV to be linked to pushing yourself beyond your limits and the fear of not being good enough, which drains all inner support, and stress. Hay associates viruses with bitterness and a lack of joy. When we take ourselves into these places, we activate this virus. This virus then wreaks havoc in our systems. EBV can be linked to the cause of many autoimmune conditions and some cancers. Why has a vaccine not being created to eradicate it? These viruses are mutating, and possibly strengthening, to be able to live in their hosts for longer periods without killing the host. Some research points to long COVID being a combination of EBV and COVID-19. If you have an autoimmune condition, it is worth checking first whether this is what is underlying all your symptoms. EBV can be pacified with diet and herbs. A plant-based diet focused on dominantly raw foods should be your first port of call here.

Coxsackievirus is another virus that causes a great deal of havoc and tends to resurface in periods of our lives where we are run down, traumatised and stressed. Chronic work or life stress, or a big shock, can trigger most dormant viruses in your system. A common culprit here is the varicella zoster virus (VZV) – the chicken pox virus – being triggered as shingles later in life. Herpes is regularly triggered by stress. Viral infections such as Herpes simplex can cause severe inflammation of brain regions, damaging neurons in the hippocampus and the temporal lobe in particular. Patients who have suffered from measles, rubella and associated viral infections may show symptoms of dementia that are subsumed under this term. An impaired autoimmune system is thought to be responsible for the underlying neuropathology. Medical practitioners rarely test for these viruses.

Viruses cause many symptoms, including migraines, depression, anxiety, brain fog, concentration issues, thyroid nodules and cysts, glaucoma, polycystic ovary syndrome (PCOS), infertility, high cholesterol, eye issues such as eye floaters, rashes, tightness in the chest, restless leg syndrome, aches and pains, arthritis, fibromyalgia, joint pain, restlessness, muscle weakness, twitches, spasms, tingles, numbness, heart palpitations, goitres, vertigo, tinnitus, body temperature issues, chronic fatigue, weak organ functioning, burning mouth, burning tongue, vaginal burning, neck pain, frozen shoulder, neuropathy, and some cancers.

Something I learnt from one of the medical practitioners I consulted is that viruses attack nerves, and that one of these nerves is the vagus nerve. When this happens, it can feel like you are being put into fight-or-flight mode, and often those with viral infections display increased anxiety. It has made me really look at the roots of those with anxiety in my practice and often I have found that this anxiety can be alleviated with a plant-based diet (by plant-based here I mean fruit and vegetables, without grains). My vagus nerve attack would result in severe mood fluctuations. I started looking at the borderline personality clients in my practice and noticed that most of them were experiencing difficulties with physical symptoms and diagnoses like fibromyalgia. It makes sense, too, that someone with a substantial trauma history would have EBV activation and that this, in part, could be driving their anxiety. Blood clotting is a common symptom of these viruses. Most viral infections deplete the body's iron reserves. So much goes out of harmony in the body, and this can have knock-on effects.

Neurotropic viruses are characterised by their ability to conceal themselves in the body, particularly in the lymph nodes and liver tissues. Neurotropic viruses can reactivate even in healthy adults, despite the fact that the initial infection may have taken place during the first ten years of life. Patients usually report symptoms of reactivation during a period of stress or illness, such as a normal cold or flu. Although latency usually occurs in neural tissue, viral infection extends to the extracellular space when it comes out of dormancy. When a neurotropic virus or any other pathogen infects the vagus nerve itself, cytokines are released directly to receptors in the sensitive vagus nerve, and this immune system becomes pathologically intense – having an effect that could look like chronic fatigue syndrome. Viruses that have an affinity for vagus nerve infection include human herpesvirus-6 (HHV-6), EBV, VZV, certain kinds of enteroviruses and even *Borrelia*.

Helicobacter pylori can enter your body and live in your digestive tract. After many years, it causes sores called ulcers in the lining of your stomach or the upper part of your small intestine. A two-week course of antibiotics is usually used to treat this, but some practitioners prefer (and you may too) taking a longer herbal remedy approach, often lasting for three months.

Start by testing for EBV, coxsackievirus, cytomegalovirus, SIBO, yeast overgrowth (especially candida) and *Helicobacter pylori*. You may want to include additional tests if you have been exposed to cats (*Bartonella*) and ticks (*Borrelia* and Lyme disease). If you test positive for these pathogens, you will need to monitor and manage your stress levels: exposure to stress and trauma is likely to reactivate infection. Each time there is a re-infection, it may create an additional layer of symptoms. Through the process of healing, these layers of symptoms generally leave in the order in which they arrived. If you have long COVID or had a difficult COVID-19 experience, it is recommended that you undergo this investigation.

Toxins

Toxins include any poisonous substance from the external environment (exotoxins), or from inside the body due to maldigestion and strained detoxification pathways (endotoxins). They are unstable substances that, when introduced to the tissues, can induce antibody formation.

Toxins can be generated by bacteria, yeast and parasites that live on or in our bodies. Disease-causing microorganisms and parasites are thus toxic in a broad sense but they are called pathogens rather than toxins. Toxins surround us and may enter our systems through food (especially in the case of processed foods), pollution (such as the quality of the air you breathe), power lines, nuclear power plants, radiation, Wi-Fi, factories, our water supply, the chemicals we use to clean our homes and wash our bodies, the makeup we wear, and many other avenues. They can be found in places you may not be considering – how healthy is it to swim in a chlorinated pool or to use air conditioning, for example? The water coming out of our taps is a very important thing to consider – in many countries the water systems are old: sometimes they are poorly maintained, and sometimes lead pipes are still in use. There is evidence that medication residues are not being filtered out of wastewater systems properly – and perhaps medications like the contraceptive pill are delivering doses of unrequired hormones. These toxins could be blocking up or weighing down your body's detoxification pathways. Tests such as liver function tests may indicate the toxic burden on your liver. Symptoms of toxicity can include nausea, diarrhoea, stomach pain, drowsiness, dizziness, weakness, high temperature, chills (shivering), loss of appetite, and headaches.

Heavy metals

Heavy metal poisoning occurs when your body's soft tissues absorb too much of a particular metal. You may be exposed to high concentrations of these metals from food, air or water pollution, as well as medicines and supplements, food containers with improper coatings, industrial exposure or lead-based paint. Heavy metal poisoning is very rare, but a heavy metal overload is more common. Symptoms of heavy metal poisoning include diarrhoea, nausea, abdominal pain, vomiting, shortness of breath, tingling in the feet and hands, chills and weakness. Blood, urine and hair tests can test for heavy metals. Heavy metals in your body and the food you consume interact with the viral content in your body, often feeding the virus residing inside you. EBV locates itself in the liver, which provides the virus with a good source of the ingredients it needs to sustain itself, as heavy metals often sit in or pass through the liver. Parasites thrive in body environments that are high in heavy metals, an environment that often reduces the effectiveness of parasite cleanses. Parasites accumulate heavy metals, and heavy metals provide a feeding ground for parasites. You can't get rid of one without working on the other. Some of the metals you may want to consider include cadmium, lead, mercury, arsenic, copper, zinc, titanium, aluminium and iron.

Mercury poisoning specifically has symptoms such as a lack of coordination, muscle weakness, hearing and speech difficulties, nerve damage in your hands and face, vision changes and trouble walking. It can take place through contaminated fish or water, X-ray machines and tooth fillings. Safely removing amalgam fillings with a biological dentist trained in this process may form part of your healing process. Fish is a healthy animal protein, but certain varieties of deep-sea fish can contain high levels of mercury as a result of this pollutant working its way up the food chain in the sea. Plants that grow in mercury-contaminated waters are consumed by small fish, which are then consumed by large fish. Mercury then accumulates in the bodies of larger fish, so larger and longer-lived fish tend to contain the most mercury – such as sharks, swordfish, fresh tuna, marlin, king mackerel, tilefish and north pike. In salmon and hake – the more popular fish – the mercury content is generally quite low. Mercury is a neurotoxin, so it can damage the brain and nerves.

Lead poisoning symptoms can include constipation, aggressive behaviour, sleep problems, irritability, high blood pressure, loss of appetite, anaemia, headache, fatigue, memory loss, and loss of developmental skills in children. Lead poisoning can occur through paint, cosmetics, hair dyes, and even through being in gun shooting ranges, which leads you to consider the possible toxicity in the environments in which you may spend time. Arsenic poisoning can take place through insecticides, contaminated seafood and contaminated water. Cadmium levels can increase as a consequence of smoking cigarettes. Copper, zinc and iron frequently occur in the daily supplements we take but there is a safe amount that the body feels comfortable with. The copper IUD contraceptive may increase copper levels in the body. Titanium and aluminium may be part of various body implants.

Food toxins

Some foods are detrimental to autoimmune conditions: refined flours (for example white bread), conventional frozen meals, white rice, microwaveable popcorn, cured meats, protein or energy bars, artificial trans fats (found in margarine, many snack foods and many baked products), soy-based products, certain types of cinnamon, refined vegetable and seed oils, plastic-packaged foods, and anything with added sugars. Unlike the oils from naturally oily foods, such as coconut oil and olive oil, vegetable and seed oils may be refined. They can produce potentially cancer-causing aldehydes, especially when used for deep frying.

A chemical in plastic containers used for food called bisphenol A (BPA) – and its newer replacement, bisphenol S (BPS) – are toxins, with BPS proving even more toxic to the reproductive system than

BPA. To avoid exposure to these compounds, avoid plastic dishware as far as possible, including bottled water, and use stainless steel drinkware instead of plastic. BPA is believed to mimic oestrogen by binding to the receptor sites meant for the hormone, which can disrupt hormone function. Oestrogen dominance has a strong link to some autoimmune conditions. BPA has also been associated in insulin resistance, type 2 diabetes and obesity. Polycyclic aromatic hydrocarbons (PAHs) are environmental pollutants that arise from burning organic material and are found in foods such as meat that is grilled or smoked at high temperatures – red meat was thought to be the main culprit here, but this is also the case with chicken. Smoked and grilled meats are the primary source of PAHs in food.

Added sugars are linked to conditions such as obesity, type 2 diabetes, fatty liver disease and cancer. Foods high in added sugars are typically also highly processed and may have addictive properties that make it harder to regulate their intake. Some researchers have attributed this addictive quality to sugar's ability to release dopamine.

Emotional toxins

Emotional toxins are toxins that arise from the interactions to which you expose yourself. Imagine that you are sitting at a restaurant and a woman suddenly comes up to you and starts shouting at you for how you parked your car. She screams numerous insults at you. Your confused and meek response is, 'I don't have a car.' She walks away without apologising. Later, when you are past the shock of the interaction, anger begins to rise up inside you. You catch yourself ruminating about this event for the rest of the day, and the next, and each time you think about it the memory could be flooding your system with anger.

From the perspective of Chinese medicine, anger affects your liver. Perhaps this push of anger causes you to wake up at the liver time of 3 a.m. Your crankiness from not sleeping plus this anger could result in your being quite reactive to others around you, so you have an argument with your partner about something minor. This is the impact of one small interaction. Consider what it means to be in a toxic relationship, where there are many of these kinds of encounters every day; think about the emotional toxins you are accumulating within.

Chemicals and radiation

An array of chemicals, radiation and other toxins drives autoimmunity. An entire book can likely be dedicated to exploring this, driven by our unnatural lifestyle. Two chemicals are very relevant, specifically for Hashimoto's. Triclosan is a chemical that is found in antibacterial soaps, deodorants, hairsprays and toothpastes. The structure of triclosan resembles the structure of thyroid hormones and has been associated with altered levels of thyroid hormone in animals. In fact, this ingredient has been banned by the US Food and Drug Administration (FDA) due to the thyroid toxicity it can cause. Fluoride, which is found in toothpaste and our water supply, lowers the pH level in the mouth, making the oral environment more acidic and thus less hospitable to bacteria. It has a negative effect on thyroid function. There is also a significant connection between radiation and thyroid autoimmunity, as has been found in people exposed to the nuclear disaster in Chernobyl. Recent studies have shown that even low doses of radiation can influence the immune system, possibly exacerbating certain autoimmune conditions such as asthma and Hashimoto's. Nuclear disasters such as Chernobyl have played a role in increasing autoimmune prevalence. I was two years old and living in Poland at the time of the Chernobyl disaster, which would have affected my developing body. Many women I know who are of Polish decent suffer from thyroid problems, and this is likely one of the drivers.

Bathroom, hygiene and beauty products are also culprits. In an average American woman's bathroom, you will likely find close to one hundred personal care products, including nail polish, lotion, shampoo, makeup remover, eyeliner, face masks, hairspray, perfume and so on. These products are full of chemicals, most of which have not undergone adequate safety studies to prove that they are not toxic. Conducting laboratory tests to assess blood levels and changes in organ or immune system function, or any other available medical tests, for that matter, are not common practice in the cosmetic industry. I needed to reconsider my use of Brazilian treatments – hair-straightening products used by hairdressers, which often contain formaldehyde – and my use of perfume and nail polish.

We need to recognise how permeable our skins are – everything you put on your skin gets absorbed. Would you eat your moisturiser or face wash? If you think about it this way, you may reconsider using it.

Implants

Breast implants have been linked to triggering autoimmune conditions. Scientists say this could be due to the fact that textured implants have a greater surface area on which a bacterial infection can form. Infections could trigger a type of immune response that ultimately leads to autoimmunity. Breast implant illness (BII) is a term that has been given to a combination of symptoms including joint and muscle pain, chronic fatigue, memory and concentration problems, breathing problems, sleep disturbance, rashes and skin problems, dry mouth and eyes, anxiety, depression, headaches, hair loss and gastrointestinal problems. Other implants may have similar effects.

Electromagnetic fields

Electromagnetic fields are something we all live in these days, with 5G Wi-Fi being available everywhere we go (www.forbes.com/health/body/is-5g-safe/). Fluorescent lights, mobile phones, Wi-Fi, cordless phones and power lines all have an impact on us, causing symptoms such as sleep disturbances, stress, fatigue, headaches, rashes, burning sensations, pain, brain fog and heart palpitations. When we start looking at every aspect of modern life, it looks like we are setting up many of these conditions for autoimmunity to flourish.

Contraception

Female contraceptive measures are a huge driver of dysregulation in women's bodies. They may not fit too neatly into this section, but they need to be discussed. Hormone-based contraceptives may dysregulate the natural balance of the hormonal system. The copper IUD causes longer menstruation, which may deplete iron reserves. Iron is necessary for the effective functioning of our immune systems.

Inflammation

Inflammation is caused by stress, trauma, pathogens, toxins and bad diet, so we can describe it as a result of some of the causes already described above, as well as a perpetuating causal factor. When you are healing, you are in essence managing chronic inflammation through addressing all the factors that cause it.

Inflammation is essential to your survival. It helps protect your body from infection and injury but can also cause severe damage and contribute to disease when it is chronic and excessive. Convincing evidence from extensive medical research indicates that the damage caused by acute inflammation often plays a dominant role in the development of many chronic diseases, including arthritis, neurological diseases and cancer.

Inflammation is a big part of autoimmune conditions, so targeting ways to lower this is a key to healing. Many types of autoimmune diseases cause redness, swelling, heat and pain, which are the signs and symptoms of inflammation. Inflammation drives the symptoms of autoimmune conditions. Several inflammatory molecules released by the immune system are also implicated in sustaining long-term, low-level inflammation, a process directly linked to autoimmunity. It is something that you want to get under control in your body – suppression of inflammation is a therapeutic strategy for the prevention and alleviation of illness.

When our bodies are overwhelmed by stress in various forms through psychological stress (past and present), the stress of infection, and the stress of toxins from our diet and environment, inflammation will arise. Foods that are pro-inflammatory include alcohol, processed meat, vegetable and seed oils (containing omega-6 fatty acids), refined carbohydrates, fried foods, red meat, margarine, added sugars, gluten and beans. With omega-3 and -6, the key is to optimise the ratio. Most people consume far too much omega-6 and it is speculated that the disrupted ratio between these fatty acid types may be one of the most damaging aspects of the Western diet. In the case of arthritis, vegetables from the nightshade family – eggplant, peppers, tomatoes and potatoes – are believed to aggravate arthritis pain and inflammation as they contain a chemical called solanine.

Our psychological health affects inflammation in our bodies, and inflammation drives our psychological health. Inflammation may play a crucial role in the development of depression. Conflict, a stressful lifestyle, fearful and worried thinking, and a lack of sleep all have a tremendous effect on increasing inflammation in the body.

Allergens

Once there is dysregulation in our ANS, we may become increasingly sensitive to the environment around us. Allergens then exacerbate the developing autoimmunity. Allergens in your environment could be stimulating your immune system and sending it into overdrive. They are developed sensitivities. Sometimes, in my practice, I have found that these are rooted in traumatic memory, as associations with a negative experience.

The main food allergens people struggle with are celery, gluten, crustaceans (such as prawns, crabs, lobsters), eggs, fish, milk, molluscs (mussels and oysters), mustard, peanuts, sesame, soybeans and sulphites. Allergens may also be environmental in that certain grasses and other plants, pollens, house dust mites, insect venoms and animal epithelial materials may create reactions. When healing from illness, it is best to use an elimination protocol to remove all these items and any others you may suspect are interfering with you for a period, then slowly reintroduce them to test which ones are problematic. You may want to remove them all for the duration of the process of your healing. Consider everything you are coming into contact with – from cleaning chemicals to the fabric of your bed sheets and, most importantly, what you are eating. There are also tests for these allergens.

At first glance, allergies and autoimmune disease may seem unrelated. But connecting the dots, we see that, in both, the immune system is reacting to something within. We don't want the immune system to flare up when it doesn't have to. When you have an autoimmune condition, it is already in overdrive, so remove everything that is bothering you as soon as possible. This may also mean looking into cosmetics and things your partner uses. Autoimmune diseases flare when they are overstimulated by various triggers. According to research, there is a significantly higher risk of autoimmunity if you have allergies, and some research has even found that autoimmunity starts with allergies. Allergens could promote the initial autoantibody development and subsequent autoimmune disease. Allergies are an initial phase of immune overstimulation that are triggered from outside of the body, whereas autoimmune reactions are a late phase of chronic immune overstimulation that occurs within the body. Both these reactions are from an exaggerated immune response.

The table that follows is from Isabella Wentz's *Hashimoto's Protocol*. These foods may be feeding the viral or bacterial load in your body, which then has an action on the various body parts or systems named on the following page:

COMMON FOOD REACTIONS	
Body system	**Symptoms**
Lungs	Postnasal drip, congestion, cough, asthma
Gut	Constipation, diarrhoea, cramping, bloating, nausea, gas, acid reflux, burning, burping
Heart	Increased pulse, palpitations
Skin	Acne, eczema, itchiness
Muscles	Joint aches, pain, swelling, tingling, numbness
Brain	Headache, dizziness, brain fog, anxiety, depression, fatigue, insomnia

Mould could also be a culprit behind your symptoms – recent research has shown that it can induce autoimmunity. It is considered an allergen, but I believe that mould exposure isn't good for anyone, even if you are not allergic to it. If you have mould in your bathroom, a stale, mouldy smell in your home, or mould on the walls of your home due to water damage, for example, you may need to clear the source of this, or even move. This is often the problem when entire families are affected by autoimmune conditions. Exclude high-mould foods and beverages, such as peanuts, raisins, dried fruit, nuts, coffee, beer and wine, from your diet.

Decreasing organ function

Our organ function is affected by our emotional state (stress and trauma), pathogens, toxins, allergens, and the resulting inflammation. This becomes a cause and a driver of autoimmunity as the system gradually deteriorates. As organ function declines, the body ceases to be able to function optimally. If you are reading this book for personal assistance, your liver may not in the best state, possibly also your gut, and certainly your adrenals. Most of my organs were not functioning optimally and I had no idea. I thought I had been taking care of myself very well with my diet, regular colonics and acupuncture. However, there was a virus attacking my liver, which was affecting my detoxification pathways; these accumulating toxins were having an effect everywhere else.

The function of an organ system depends on the integrated activity of all other organs in the body. The major organs to look at are the following:

- Brain: Controls the body (look at things like memory, attention, seizures, neurological things going on in the body, your mood/emotions, etc.)
- Eyes: Control vision
- Heart: Circulates blood
- Kidneys: Excrete water and waste products
- Lungs: Supply oxygen to the blood
- Liver: Removes waste created by digestion
- Skin: Excretes waste, forms an external protective coating
- Stomach: Digests food
- Colon: Absorbs nutrients from food, processes waste
- Spleen: Important for the immune system and filtering blood
- Nerves: Transmit information and signals around the body
- Blood: Moves oxygen and nutrition around the body.

The three organs to focus on when initiating your healing journey are your liver, gut and adrenals. Issues in these set the body up for a cascade of events that result in the autoimmune condition. Your liver function affects the detoxification of your body. Your gut function affects detoxification and nutrient absorption. I have already discussed adrenaline extensively, so you've seen how overactive adrenals suppress your immune system. What rating would you give right now to your liver, intestinal and adrenal function, out of ten?

Fatty liver

The liver plays a key role in detoxifying the system. Our livers are hard workers in a modern age full of environmental toxins. Environmental factors can be compounded by substance abuse and unhealthy food choices. Whether you eat something, inhale it, or put it on your skin, it will go into your bloodstream and your liver will need to process it.

It takes about three to ten days to move alcohol and drugs out of an addict's system, a good gauge for estimating how long it would take the liver to let go of what it needs to. Symptoms of toxic build-up include chronic digestive issues, fatigue, anxiety and depression, skin issues, muscle and joint aches and pains, cravings, insomnia, blood sugar imbalances, bad breath and foul-smelling stool.

Fatty liver may occur as a consequence of inflammation from a virus, medication, alcohol or diet (the liver doesn't do well with deep-fried food, for example). Certain over-the-counter medications like aspirin, as well as a popular cholesterol medication, have a strong impact on the liver. Most medications strain the liver somewhat. Over time, as the liver becomes damaged, fat replaces it. It is difficult to detect the extent of liver damage through blood tests, so you need to do a biopsy. You can also develop scar tissue in the liver, which leads to cirrhosis. The liver is an amazing organ, and you can get away with even a small portion of the liver working properly. When the liver swells up, there can be heart arrythmia issues, skipped heart beats, high blood pressure and a compressed heart. The liver can completely regenerate; however, the process takes a long time (up to three years). It is important to stop the things that are damaging your liver and begin to add those that aid regeneration.

Leaky gut

If you have an autoimmune or trauma-driven condition your gut lining is likely eroded, and an imbalance of bacteria is likely at play. As you've seen, we call this leaky gut. Intestinal permeability results in the intestinal barrier being impaired, allowing toxins into your bloodstream and creating inflammation all over your body.

Typically, the digestive tract allows for selective permeability, which only lets digested food particles though. In leaky gut, the passage of not only normally digested nutrient building blocks (amino acids, fatty acids and simple sugars from carbohydrates), but also larger food particles (larger-chain proteins, fats and carbohydrates, and toxins that were never meant to pass through) is allowed. This weakens and overstimulates the immune system. We can liken this to a screen on a window. If the screen is functioning properly and has no holes in it, air will pass through, but flies, mosquitoes and other bugs will not. But if the screen has tears in it, making larger holes, all types of insects will get through it.

While there are numerous causes of intestinal permeability, the most common ones are stress, food sensitivities, nutrient deficiencies, deficiency in digestive enzymes, an imbalance of gut bacteria, and intestinal infections. Intestinal permeability explains the regularly appearing gut symptoms in autoimmune conditions such as bloating, stomach pain, IBS, acid reflux, nutritional deficiencies, headaches, difficulty concentrating, joint pain, skin problems and widespread inflammation.

Adrenal fatigue

All stress accumulates in the body, even the stress of birth. Your adrenals are reacting now, in the present time, to the many stressful events that have happened over the course of your life. It is as if you have too many applications running on your desktop, using energy from your adrenals – making your adrenals function improperly.

Adrenal fatigue results, which is directly related to the HPA axis we discussed earlier. You'll recall that this is the pathway that manages our response to stress and the release of cortisol, and that it is triggered when our body encounters a stressful stimulus. Usually, the stimulus is short-lived. The hypothalamus signals the pituitary gland to release hormones that affect the adrenal glands, which subsequently produce cortisol. Finally, cortisol travels through the body to respond to the stimulus. Cortisol and other glucocorticoids also manage the inflammatory response by upregulating anti-inflammatory signals and downregulating pro-inflammatory chemicals. The result is suppression of the immune system.

Adrenal fatigue can be the result of chronic stress on the body due to an external stressor, such as a stressful work environment, relationship stress, or family stress, or an underlying cause of stress on the body, such as a chronic infection or chronic disease like an autoimmune disease. When the adrenals are overtaxed and become exhausted, symptoms may include fatigue, exercise and stress intolerance, insomnia, metabolic disturbances, frequent infections, heart palpitations and hypoglycaemia. The effects of a weak adrenal system are therefore felt throughout the body. Alternative theories on the concept of 'adrenal fatigue' exist, in that it is not the adrenals that actually tire out, but rather that the brain, becoming averse to constantly high cortisol, begins to downregulate cortisol production to protect itself, so it's more that the adrenals are 'turned down' than fatigued. Whichever way we look at it, it is useful and necessary to understand the impact of the adrenals in these conditions.

Autoimmunity on a cellular level

Diving a bit deeper into the body, on a cellular level autoimmunity can be linked to mitochondrial dysfunction. Mitochondria are the parts of our cells that convert the energy of food molecules into the energy format that powers most of our bodily functions, like breathing, digestion and our immune system. They play a big role in protection from disease and the ageing process.

According to a review published in the journal *Molecular Cell*, mitochondria also play a role in supporting your immune system and cellular signalling when the body is under stress. Like plants turn carbon dioxide into oxygen, our mitochondria take the glucose from food and make adenosine triphosphate (ATP). When the mitochondria cease to do their jobs properly, fatigue is the first result, since the mitochondria produce over 90 per cent of the usable energy in the body. After that, symptoms affect the parts of the body that require the highest amount of ATP. These include the brain, muscles, heart, liver, lungs, kidneys and GI tract. Mitochondrial functionality appears to be very sensitive to environmental toxins such as pesticides. In other words, exposure to toxins, even commonly used pesticides, may affect your mitochondrial health and increase your risk of developing certain chronic health conditions. This discovery is providing a promising pathway to treating the autoimmune problem.

Out-of-balance energetic system

Your body is an energetic system that has a frequency. The energy that you put in, is the energy you resonate out. Everything you eat, the activities you do and the people you engage with contribute to tuning your frequency. Others get drawn to you (or repelled by you) based on this frequency. People take on your frequency and you take on those of others. Looking after your energetic system may mean eating lots of raw, fresh foods full of life-giving vibration, spending time with high-energy/vibration people, and engaging in high-vibration activities.

The ancient medicine traditions all have concepts of the energy system woven into their foundations. Often, this energy system is also deeply connected to the spirituality in the system. Yogic and ayurvedic traditions talk about the chakra system. TCM speaks about *qi*, vital energy or material energy. Even tribes in the Amazon like the Shipibo use ayahuasca to diagnose difficulties as energy blockages, excess energy or where energy is lacking. They diagnose where negative, dense energies are trapped in the system and work, guided by plant spirits, to cleanse and purify the body of these energies. They understand that negative energy is not native to our bodies and that it can control the way we think, the way we perceive and the way we experience life. It blocks the flow of positive energy, affecting our ability to connect with ourselves and others, and holds us back from reaching our true potential.

Autoimmunity can be looked at as an energy disruption. Your energetic system becomes stuck in an unwell configuration, and this is why it is so difficult to shift without addressing all the moving parts. Your body has taken on a frequency of sickness, forgetting where its alignment is, and we need to remind it about who you are so that all the healing modalities you are engaging with have a chance to be effective. Perhaps it starts with the more psychology-based causes that disrupt the body energetically, then solidifies in physiology. Many energy practitioners are able to locate energy imbalances long before they manifest in a physical outcome. Energy healing may be a necessary stop on this healing journey to remind your body of its healthy resonance.

An effective way of diagnosing your energetic system is to look at your chakras. The chakras are spinning energy vortices, energy points in your body. There are seven main chakras located along your spine. These energy points should stay 'open' and aligned, as they correspond to major organs and systems that affect our physical and emotional well-being.

Diagnosis using the chakra system includes looking at your physical medical history and emotional history, and indicating where your imbalance is housed. There could be a depletion of energy flow, or too much energetic activity in a chakra, and each will manifest in different outcomes. When a chakra is low in energy, you may have difficulty expressing the particular qualities associated with that chakra. When a chakra is overactive, the qualities are a dominant – sometimes overpowering – force in your life. This can have both physical and emotional effects.

In general, the location of the chakra that is out of balance may affect the parts of your body in close proximity to that chakra – the organs, bones, joints and tissues near that area. Psychologically, imbalances in the chakras may cause increased anger, sadness, fear or indecisiveness. Experiencing too much stress – physically or mentally – may cause one or more chakras to be out of balance. Personal habits such as poor physical alignment or posture, eating unhealthy food, or self-destructive behaviour may cause a chakra to become imbalanced. Prolonged imbalance may lead to physical disease and illness.

Again, I recommend reading *Eastern Body, Western Mind* by Anodea Judith, and much of Caroline Myss, to assist you in finding alignment here. When balanced, our chakras contribute to immune system health and the body's ability to heal itself. When any of the chakras are blocked or out of balance, the immune system suffers. Homeostasis, in which the body's various parts work together to maintain health, is highly dependent on balanced chakras and free energy flow. The immune system, then, can be conditioned and nourished through proper care of the chakras. The future of medicine likely lies in containing and concentrating the powerful healing that lies in energetic and frequency-based modalities such as acupuncture, yoga, homeopathy and other vibrational modalities in combination with technology to directly affect our out-of-balance energy systems.

PART 3

Solutions: What can you do about it?

To HEAL FROM and manage autoimmune and other trauma-driven conditions, you are going to need to engage with a variety of healing methods and practitioners. Each layer of healing will require you to exercise agency over your own lifestyle and create your own wellness protocols to regulate yourself and bring your body back to its default healthy setting. Various practitioners will resonate with you at different points in the process.

Ensure that you are nourishing your body, and not punishing it, through this process. In our desperation to get better, we may try rush and push the process (especially those Type A personalities). Listen to what your body needs and go slowly. This can be financially taxing too, so go at a pace that doesn't create added pressure.

We need to let go of previous routines and allow ourselves to engage spontaneously using the felt sense and wisdom in our bodies. According to some eastern traditions, when you need to make a decision, you swallow it. You then allow the body to feel it, and you listen to what comes through the body to guide you.

Healing practitioners

An important part of your journey will be to enlist the support of practitioners who are experienced in the various aspects of yourself that will need work. This section contains some of the modalities I recommend. I have listed the most vital practitioners first: I recommend starting with an integrative (or functional) medical doctor and a somatic or trauma-based psychologist, as well as one adjunct alternative method.

Integrative or functional medicine

Our society is experiencing a sharp increase in the number of people who are suffering from complex, chronic diseases, such as diabetes, heart disease, cancer, mental illness and autoimmune disorders. The system of medicine practised by most physicians is oriented towards acute care: the diagnosis and treatment of trauma or illness that is of short duration and in need of urgent care, such as appendicitis or a broken leg. Physicians apply specific, prescribed treatments such as drugs or surgery that aim to treat the immediate problem or symptom. Often, medication is prescribed specifically to manage certain symptoms, but this does not address the issue from a long-term perspective. Many of those with autoimmune conditions are also sensitive to medications, which often have adverse side effects. Some of the traditional practices in treating autoimmune conditions, like destroying part of the thyroid in Graves' disease, may actually be counterproductive in terms of the balance of the body. In another situation, a client I worked with found near complete relief from his condition in the surgical removal of part of his gut, so there is certainly value in traditional medical interventions for some.

Unfortunately, the acute-care approach to medicine often lacks the proper methodology and tools for preventing and treating complex, chronic disease. In most cases, it does not consider the unique genetic makeup of each individual or factors such as environmental exposures to toxins, mental health and the aspects of today's lifestyle that have a direct influence on the rise of chronic disease in modern western society. There is an enormous gap between emerging research in basic sciences and integration into medical practice – as long as fifty years – particularly in the area of complex, chronic illness. Most physicians are not adequately trained to assess the underlying causes of complex, chronic disease and to apply strategies such as nutrition, diet, lifestyle and exercise to treat and prevent these illnesses in their patients. A new type of practice has emerged from this gap, called integrative or functional medicine.

Integrative or functional medicine is healing-oriented medicine that takes account of the whole person (body, mind and spirit), including all aspects of lifestyle. It is an investigative approach that takes the whole history of the individual into account, recognising that no two individuals are the same. It looks at the body in its entirety, understanding the interconnectedness between each organ. It looks not only at symptoms, but also at how emotions and stress are affecting the body. It emphasises the therapeutic relationship and makes use of all appropriate therapies, both conventional and alternative. In other words, integrative medicine 'cherry picks' the very best, scientifically validated therapies from both conventional and alternative systems. It is a system that recognises that to heal you may need a team of practitioners who focus on different areas. It is also a system that encourages the individual's choice and agency.

This systems-biology-based approach focuses on identifying and addressing the root cause of disease. It addresses issues layer by layer, in a gradual manner, getting to ever-deeper roots. It considers genetic vulnerabilities and uses nutrition, lifestyle and supplements based on these to ameliorate progression. It determines which pathways in our body may not working effectively (e.g. detoxification, iron absorption, vitamin B metabolism) and designs a treatment plan to address this.

Each symptom or differential diagnosis may be one of many contributing to an individual's illness. A diagnosis can result from multiple causes, which is illustrated in the diagram that follows. For instance, inflammation is just one of the many factors that could contribute to depression. Likewise, a cause such as inflammation may lead to a number of different diagnoses, including depression. The precise manifestation of each cause depends on the individual's genes, environment and lifestyle, and only treatments that address the right cause will have lasting benefits beyond symptom suppression.

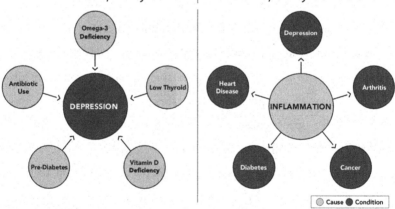

Used with permission from The Institute for Functional Medicine (IFM), the global leader in functional medicine and a collaborator in the transformation of healthcare.

Functional medicine treats the whole person, not just a discrete group of symptoms, by shifting from the traditional disease-centred focus of medical practice to a more patient-centred approach. Practitioners in functional medicine invest time in getting to know their patients, learning about their histories, and analysing how interactions between genetic, environmental and lifestyle factors may affect complex, chronic disease and long-term health. Functional medicine encourages each person's individual manifestation of health and vitality in this way. The focus is on prevention through nutrition or diet and exercise; use of the latest laboratory testing and other diagnostic techniques; and prescribed combinations of drugs and/or botanical medicines, supplements, therapeutic diets, detoxification programmes, or stress-management techniques.

If you have one of those medical doctors who sees you for ten minutes and sends you off with a script for medication, you need to change doctors. Find a doctor who makes an effort to learn about you and your life. One who is willing to dig through your blood work and find the patterns and connections that others don't see – someone who spends time understanding your body, your lifestyle, your mental health and your family history. A person who is able to follow the allopathic route and perhaps also the herbal, diet and supplement route with solutions for your body and your mind. A person who is willing and able to work with other practitioners, should it be required. It is vital that they are trauma conscious, recognising that this is a contributing causal factor. Not someone who runs up medical bills by sending you for incessant unnecessary testing and screening, but someone who can provide support and solutions.

Psychology
Somatic and trauma-based methods of psychotherapy

Psychotherapy is a must, especially at the beginning of your health difficulties, if only to have an external pillar of strength to keep you going. You need support; you need to feel safe and not alone in this. At a later stage, when you are ready, psychotherapy will also need to guide you in determining how this illness has been manifested and help you work through the deeper patterns of trauma that underlie and are likely to maintain it. Trauma work is a necessity to get your mind under control so that it can be clear-thinking and present, and so that you can stop being your own cortisol volcano. Through trauma work, you also trauma-proof yourself.

I recommend somatic psychotherapy for trauma processing. Talk therapy is simply not enough when the body is stuck in a dysregulated state. The body needs to shake, cry, vibrate, scream, twitch the trauma out. We need to do limbic system therapy, to calm down the amygdala that is flaring out of control. When we work somatically with trauma, we work with its root cause. We don't work directly with symptoms, such as anxiety or autoimmune conditions. The aim is to resolve the symptoms, rather than merely find ways to cope with them.

According to somatic therapy theory, the sensations associated with past trauma may become trapped within the body and reflected in facial expressions, posture, muscular pain, or other forms of body language. A chronically overstimulated nervous system requires a type of psychotherapy process that focuses on releasing the stored and stuck energy of complex trauma. The mind affects the body as we tend to hold unresolved emotional trauma in the tissues. Somatic psychotherapy is the most effective approach for autoimmune conditions in that it is focused on regulating traumatic experiences out of the system. This type of therapy depends on the bodily experiences of the individual as a gateway to re-experiencing the traumatic event in a safe environment and carrying out any previously unfulfilled actions to achieve a feeling of completion and closure. Details of the trauma do not necessarily need to be recalled for the treatment to be effective.

Emotions have a direct effect on how the body works. Negative emotions stimulate the glandular system for the release of harmful chemicals (hormones) while positive emotions release useful chemicals, also in the form of hormones. As we've seen, if negative emotions persist in the psyche for a long time, they can affect the body's chemical balance and other systems, such as the immune and endocrine systems. In psychology, Freud came up with the term 'abreaction', which is in essence a purge of emotional excesses. 'Catharsis' was another word – the process of releasing repressed emotion. Somewhere along the way this got lost, and psychotherapy was sidetracked to the cognitive and oriented towards coping with emotions rather than releasing them. Somatic psychotherapy returns us to the process of releasing.

Psychotherapy should include a few layers of healing often occurring simultaneously:

- *Working through triggers to access unconscious trauma memory.* We want to process the traumatic memory to the end, so that we can change the way it is stored in your brain and become wisdom, instead of a background avalanche of emotions that gets triggered every time there is an associative activator (a reminder) in the present environment. Triggers may cause reactive emotions that lead us to say things we regret, act out in self-destructive and self-defeating ways, throw tantrums, sulk, indulge in addictions, make idle promises, withdraw, gossip, blame, project and manipulate, use physical violence or go numb. Becoming aware and working through our triggers can allow us to be more emotionally regulated.

- *Creating consciousness of the repeating patterns from your past.* By identifying and reprocessing these emotional patterns and belief systems, you can work through the history of what happened and reshape it into a new pattern. This in turn allows for constructive change and forward movement into an empowered solution, which aligns with your sense of purpose and authentic self. Resolving our patterns stops the domino effect of repeating the trauma from our past, in the present. For example, we no longer get drawn to controlling, abusive men, as we have worked through the roots of this pattern as something rooted in our relationship with the first man in our lives – our father.

- *Understanding your projections to release you from repeating patterns of your past in your present.* Projection means I see the world as it is, and then I add something to it – I view the world through the lens of my previous life experiences. We carry into every experience a projection based on our history of similar experiences. We see a woman with red hair and all of a sudden, we have a giggly, excited feeling as though we are twelve years old again, and we carry that energy with us through the next few hours, making life feel quite pleasant. That red-haired woman was perhaps a trigger of silly memories of your red-haired best friend at that young age on a subconscious level. Those memories may not have come up into your consciousness, but the feelings sure did. This is how we operate all the time. Now, imagine you are someone who hasn't had an easy time in life. Perhaps that red-haired woman is associated with an abusive teacher or a girl who stole your doll when you were three years old (something you likely don't remember consciously at all, as story memory for such events is not adequately developed yet at that age). How you behave towards red-haired women is then the projection that you need to become aware of. Understanding other people's projections may also be useful as a protective, trauma-proofing measure to help you stay rooted in who you are, no longer being flung around by others' perceptions of you. Often, this will allow you to reconnect with others – and yourself.

- *Somatically processing the trauma memories to re-regulate the autonomic nervous system.* This means that release happens on three levels: cognitively through speaking, emotionally through feeling, and physically through the body's discharge of trauma. As we regulate each trauma out of the body, our physiological state will change and various faculties that have got stuck in the trauma will come back online again.

- *Increasing resilience.* This means increasing vagal tone or widening our window of tolerance. This allows us to develop greater resilience in our functioning and expands what we can handle in our daily lives. Vagal tone can be increased by safely (and successfully) experiencing challenging situations and becoming aware of the resources we have inside us to do so.

- *Resolving the coping personality that you acquired in childhood that maintains your autoimmune condition.* Through conditional love and role reversal (where children take responsibility and become the parents), coping personalities are formed and our true identity gets somewhat lost. The last layer of healing will be to work with the coping personality to move into a space of clear boundaries and self-assertion. The process will bring you to your authentic self. To get here, you are going to need to give yourself the unconditional love you did not receive in childhood. For the autoimmune personality this means moving away from being Type A, from being overly responsible, and from emotional suppression, rigidity or pleasing (among others).

There are many different methods of somatic psychotherapy. I use an integrative approach that uses both somatic and relational psychodynamic elements. My recommendation is to start with Somatic Experiencing (SE) or something similar. This therapy is very effective for autoimmune conditions – it offers the titration that is necessary to avoid overwhelming an already overwhelmed body. It was originally developed by Peter Levine for the treatment of PTSD. It is a therapy that addresses autonomic dysregulation, benefiting patients who have intense overactivation, such as rage, terror or panic, or underactivation, such as emptiness and numbness. It works with interoception (a lesser-known sense that helps you understand and feel what's going on inside your body) and small increments of triggers of the patient's traumas, with alternating comforting experiences. Here are some SE terms to get you familiar with aspects of this therapeutic approach:

- Resources: Discovering what's right with the client (their strengths) and using that information to develop an inventory of resources to help the client access a sense of safety or support that can help neutralise overarousal when it comes up during sessions. This may include harnessing the power of physical resources – for example, finding the experience of being grounded or safe in the body.

- Felt sense: Helping clients develop a sensate focus and ability to track their experiences in the body. The key here is reconnecting the client to their body, and experiencing how emotions feel in the body.

- Pendulation: This involves switching between resourcing and titration, moving a person between a state of working through a traumatic memory, then back into a state of safety. This assists clients in digesting overwhelming material without becoming overwhelmed.

- Pacing: Learning the slower rate and rhythm needed to integrate traumatic material when including the physiological reorganisation. 'Slow is fast and less is more' in the service of effective integration, as the trauma brain processes much slower than our rational, logical brain regions.

- Titration: Breaking the activation down into small enough pieces to be integrated easily so that a client can process overwhelming material in a way that is not re-traumatising.

- Discharge: Supporting discharge of residual arousal in the autonomic nervous system, including completion of defensive responses that originated at the time of trauma.

The key to health is to start carefully exploring and expressing blocked emotions, and thus complete the unfinished emotional process. Doing so will change our feelings, our behaviours and the internal workings of our body. The body narrative needs to be heard, perhaps even before the verbal narrative or interpretation. Memories should be worked with directly, resources identified, and corrective shifts made that lead to a new feeling experience in the body – one that allows for the felt sense of safety. I recommend reading Bessel van der Kolk's *The Body Keeps the Score,* as well as Peter Levine's *In an Unspoken Voice* to introduce yourself to psychotherapy for trauma.

A good adjunct to the psychotherapy process is using Trauma Release Exercises (TRE). This is a method created by David Berceli that uses yoga-like positions to activate a natural reflex of shaking or vibrating in the body. This reflex helps to release deep muscular patterns of stress, tension, anxiety and trauma. TRE can calm the nervous system and restore a state of balance. With severe trauma, I recommend using this tool in the presence of a practitioner in a safe, controlled environment. However, most of us may feel comfortable in being guided by the book and doing it independently.

✎ Task

I always ask people to write down their life story at the start of psychotherapy. It is an important part of opening the pain inside us so that it can come into the light to heal. Write down your life story – with a focus on all the bad, distressing, embarrassing, humiliating things that happened at every age of your life. This reveals the memories you need to work with – the start of those memories, at least as many others lift through the psychotherapy process in a scaffolded manner. It is as though the psyche gets stronger as we work and grows the means to confront deeper and more difficult patterns. Pull out all the 'I am not safe' and 'I am alone' memories to help with your reconnection to others. We need to reset your triggers so that your emotions are no longer the source of your flare-ups. This will change the way you relate to this world – your boundaries, your coping strategies, and the essence of who you feel you are.

Find a therapist who resonates with you, preferably someone who understands autoimmune conditions. Working with autoimmune conditions in psychotherapy is often a stop-and-start event – your therapist needs to gauge where you are in every session and move gently not overexpose you to emotions that will cause excessive flare-ups. Flare-ups are inevitable, however, and you will need to manage these as you work. These flare-ups will have a different quality from normal ones – they will feel like there has been a working through.

When you are in the process of psychotherapy, be gentle with yourself. Long baths, warm herbal teas, hugs, gentle walks in nature, supportive friends (if accessible) and time with animals seem to do the trick. If you find you cannot tolerate working directly with the trauma, there are kinesiologists and energy healers out there who are gifted enough to work with the trauma in your energy field, and this may provide some relief. When you are stronger, you can again attempt a psychotherapy approach to work with regulating the trauma out of your nervous system.

Family constellations

Often, when I am sitting with a psychotherapy patient, I wish I could have a conversation with the patient's family members and sometimes even reprimand them. Family members are often not amenable to this, as the patient in my room is the black sheep to be treated and the family dynamics that led them to this place are not considered.

Family constellations is an approach to revealing and healing your underlying family patterns. It reveals the hidden dynamics beneath the surface of your relationships and allows you to work through them without the need for the family members to be present. Through this deeper understanding, it can allow negative constrictive patterns of relationship to move into more healthy life affirming patterns of the relationship. It allows you to free yourself from the damaging repetitive patterns, behaviours and emotions that are limiting your life in some way, which you have unconsciously taken on from your family system. It works with physical, energetic and emotional force fields, which become visible through representatives of human relatives or topics.

In this modality, a group of people comes together to imitate the family situation. Powerful emotions may surface during the process, so it is important to be ready for this. Give yourself time to integrate after each session. If you don't want to do this in a group, there are practitioners who do individual work and use placeholders or themselves as family members.

Craniosacral therapy

Craniosacral therapy (CST) uses a light touch to work with the membranes and fluids of the central nervous system (CNS). The craniosacral system consists of the fluid and membranes of the brain and spinal cord. It is becoming increasingly well known for its comprehensive range of therapeutic effects and its ability to align the skull and spine, balancing the autonomic functioning of the nervous system. When our bodies compensate for the everyday stress they experience, our tissues can tighten and affect the craniosacral system, which affects the way in which the nervous system functions. CST practitioners use gentle touch to release the restrictions in areas where cerebrospinal fluid cannot move around freely. This is a perfect therapy for those with autoimmune conditions, where the body is often highly sensitive to any input. Relieving tension in the CNS promotes a feeling of well-being by eliminating pain and boosting health and immunity.

CST is increasingly being used as a preventive health measure for its ability to bolster resistance to disease and is effective for a wide range of medical problems associated with pain and dysfunction. You may feel a decrease in pain or an increase in function immediately after the session, or the effects may develop gradually over the next few days. You may also experience a reorganisation phase as your body releases previously held patterns and adapts to a new state of wellness.

CST is also a very effective treatment for trauma as it re-regulates the ANS and can change psychological patterns by accessing unconscious body trauma and shifting it out of the system. In times when you do not have the energy to talk in psychotherapy, or when you do not know what to talk about, this is a very good alternative.

Massage

Massage is the application of pressure to ease pain and tension, but it is also more than that – it is a transfer of energy from one person to another. I recommend, if resources allow, that you have regular massages during your healing period – even daily, to start.

Massage helps cleanse the lymphatic system, aiding in

detoxification. Sometimes, people who deal with chronic pain have heightened sensitivity and react badly to more aggressive forms of body therapy, so choose something gentle as a start. Some benefits of massage include reducing stress and increasing relaxation, reducing pain, muscle soreness and tension, improving circulation, energy, and alertness, lowering heart rate and blood pressure, increasing joint flexibility, and reducing headache and migraine pain. Massage can help RA, MS and fibromyalgia by reducing pain, depression and anxiety, and decreasing inflammation. In Ayurveda, massage is used to detox and to recalibrate the natural rhythms of the body.

In a study looking at the effects of massage, participants had lower cytokine levels. Massage was also found to have an effect on participants' hormone levels, increasing oxytocin levels and decreasing levels of cortisol and vasopressin, a hormone believed to play a role in aggressive behaviour. Studies also suggest that massages may benefit the immune system. In one particular research study, it was shown that people who received massages had an increased number of natural killer cells and lymphocytes, white blood cells that play a large role in defending the body from disease. Lymphatic vessels are critical for clearing fluid and inflammatory cells from inflamed tissues and have roles in immune tolerance. There is a functional association of the lymphatics with the immune system, and lymphatic dysfunction may contribute to the physiology of autoimmune diseases. Therapies such as massage and acupuncture may be useful in improving lymphatic function in autoimmune diseases. Remember to drink lots of water or herbal tea before and after a massage as it can shift toxins in the body, and you want these to have an easy flow out of your system.

Reflexology

Dating back to ancient China and Egypt, reflexology involves applying pressure to the feet, hands and outer ears. It heals through deep relaxation, reduces pain and results in stronger nerve stimulation. As the diagram that follows shows, reflexology points are linked to various organs and organ systems. Stimulating these points has a balancing and detoxifying effect on the body's systems.

People who have autoimmune conditions could find reflexology helpful through detoxification and increased balance in the digestive system, immune system, respiratory system and endocrine system. Reflexology triggers parasympathetic activation, which lowers stress hormones and has healing and relaxing effects. The kidneys and liver can be directly targeted to aid the breakdown of unnecessary products in the body, which can then be cleared out. You can also learn the reflexology points and self-administer this form of treatment.

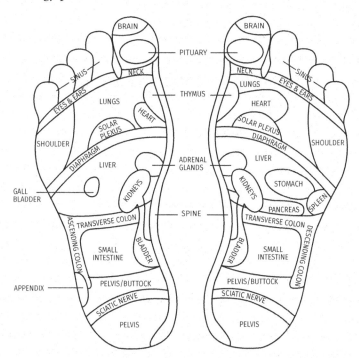

Traditional Chinese medicine (TCM)

TCM typically consists of two components – acupuncture and herbal formulas – although diet, massage, physical exercise and meditation are also known to form part of it. Diagnosis in TCM is highly individualised. Once the practitioner has identified an impaired organ system and/or emotional imbalance, he or she uses the patient's unique symptoms to determine the treatment approach. TCM considers the flow of energy, or *qi* and *xue*, in the body.

The main organs that TCM considers are the liver, kidney, heart, lungs and spleen. The organs and emotions are linked in TCM, with imbalances in the liver equating to anger, kidneys with fear, lungs with grief and sadness, spleen with worry, and heart with joy. For example, according to TCM theory, excessive irritability and anger can affect the liver and result in multiple ailments, including menstrual pain, breast distention, headaches, redness of the face and eyes, dizziness and a dry mouth. The reverse is possible in that imbalances in the liver can result in irritability and stormy moods. The liver ensures that energy and blood flow smoothly throughout the body. It also regulates bile secretion and stores blood, and is connected with the tendons, nails and eyes. The liver looks after the flow of *qi* around the body and the storage of *xue*.

An increasing number of studies have demonstrated that acupuncture treatment can control immune modulation. Acupuncture works on aligning your energetic system, and energy medicine is core medicine. Traditionally, acupuncture involves the insertion of thin needles through your skin, but for those who are sensitive to pain there is an option that involves the use of a red light instead of needles.

According to TCM, the presence of an autoimmune condition indicates causes that lie at a deep energetic level and that are different from a pathogen infection. The immune dysfunction also indicates a pathology of the Yin aspects of the immune system – Blood, bone marrow and Kidneys. TCM explains autoimmune conditions as Latent Heat and Yin Fire. There is an interesting common feature of some autoimmune diseases, which is the pulse. In TCM, it is described as having the quality of leather – superficial and stretched, like a drum, but empty at the deep level. The leather pulse indicates severe deficiency of Blood, Essence, or Yin. It also indicates *qi* floating upwards because it is not rooted by Blood. This would indicate that the root of these autoimmune diseases is a kidney deficiency. Consider that kidneys are associated with the emotions of fear in TCM, and thus the emotional link to trauma.

If this is all going over your head, let the practitioners do what they do to deal with it. It may help to talk to them about how they understand what is going on in your body, as gaining an understanding here may help you maintain your own balance in the future.

TCM describes the various conditions as follows, for example:
- Sjögren's syndrome: Yin Xu of Stomach and Liver
- Hashimoto's thyroiditis: Phlegm, Spleen-Qi Xu, Kidney-Yang Xu
- Crohn's disease: Damp-Heat in Intestines
- MS: Dampness, Stomach-Spleen Xu, Liver-Kidneys Xu
- RA: Damp-Heat in joints

To address autoimmune conditions, TCM believes that you must treat the kidneys. This can be Kidney-Yang, Kidney-Yin, Jing, Yuan Qi or Minister Fire. Secondly, inflammation must be treated with at least one or two anti-inflammatory herbs. Lastly, the practitioner should check if there is Latent Heat or Yin Fire and treat them accordingly.

There are formulations in TCM that can assist with autoimmune conditions. Some of these are available in health shops and online on websites such as China Herb. I recommend consulting with a TCM practitioner before using these herbs.

Homeopathy

Homeopathy is a system that uses tiny amounts of natural substances, like plants and minerals, to help stimulate the healing process in the body. The basic belief behind homeopathy is that 'like cures like' – something that brings on the symptoms in a healthy person can treat the illness. When you attend a homeopath, communicate as much as possible about your present symptoms and present experience in life: something as strange as having a recently acquired craving for pickles, for example, could help the homeopath to finding the right remedy or combination of remedies for you. Homeopathy is yet another way to balance the biochemistry. There are remedies that can assist with every symptom that autoimmunity brings. The homeopath is, in essence, the modern potion-maker, and there is certainly something magical about it.

Bach flower remedies are often considered similar to homeopathy, in that small amounts of natural substances are used to treat body and mind. Bach flower remedies are especially useful in the case of the psychological and emotional aspects of autoimmune conditions. These are solutions of brandy and water than contain dilutions of flower material. The belief behind them is that they can cure emotional problems by restoring the balance between mind and body and releasing suppressed negative emotions. There are 38 different remedies. Remedies are selected based on the type of person you are and the emotional experiences you are having. Crab apple and beech are useful remedies for Type A personalities where there is too much focus on perfectionism. Pine is a good remedy for those with a tendency to blame themselves. Star of Bethlehem is a useful remedy in processing shock and trauma.

Ayurveda

At about 5 000 years old, Ayurveda is the believed to be the oldest form of medicine, having its roots in India and surrounds. It harnesses the mind–body connection to promote longevity.

In Ayurveda, treatment is focused on balancing the doshas, or constitutional types. It is believed that, when there is an imbalance of the doshas, poor health can result. There are three main doshas: kapha (or water), vata (or air) and pitta (or fire). Most individuals have one dominant dosha but may also be a combination of these.

There are physical and emotional characteristics of each of these types. The vata dosha is the force behind all movements, including nerve impulses, peristalsis, the movement of thoughts, the blinking of the eyes, the heartbeat and the circulation of blood. Vata types tend to be thin and have a hard time gaining weight; tend to have light-brown hair, dry skin and delicate features; prefer sour or salty foods and may develop constipation easily; and tend to be hyperactive but have poor endurance. The pitta dosha controls digestion, metabolism and energy production. The primary function of pitta is transformation. Those with a predominance of the pitta principle have a fiery nature that manifests in both body and mind. Pitta types are of medium build with well-developed muscles; tend to be athletic and goal-oriented; prefer sweet and raw foods; and often develop inflammatory diseases. The kapha dosha represents structure, grounding and stability as the energy it carries gives substance and support to our physical body. It hydrates all the cells in our body, lubricates the joints, and maintains and protects the tissues. Kapha types tend to be short and stocky; have round features and tend to have a sluggish metabolism; prefer pungent or bitter foods, and do not like a lot of spices; and may be prone to respiratory illnesses. There is plenty to say about each of these types and you can investigate this further for yourself should you wish to.

Panchakarma is an Ayurvedic detoxification programme that systematically removes toxic burdens from both the body and mind slowly and gradually to avoid damaging the body. It is usually quite a gentle and careful process, but there are moments of intensity. During the process, you can witness how emotion is stored in the body as deeper levels of detoxification liberate trapped emotion.

Therapies in Ayurveda include herbal medicines, special diets, meditation, yoga, massage, laxatives, enemas and medical oils. These medical oils are often blended with herbs and are very powerful in treating the body, both internally and externally. A variety of techniques are used in Ayurvedic treatment. The specific technique of shirodhara, for example, includes pouring milk or oil over the forehead in the form of regular stream from a specific height in a fixed form of oscillatory movements. This is believed to act on the pituitary gland and pineal gland. It is a very effective treatment for anxiety, worry, depression, sleeplessness (due to it stimulating melatonin release) and trauma (as it normalises serotonin and noradrenaline levels in the brain). This may have an action on the HPA axis, helping us regulate our derailed adrenals and neurotransmitters. This is a very important treatment in re-regulating the ANS, and is pivotal in autoimmune treatment.

In texts that are over 5 000 years old, Ayurveda mentions conditions that have the same symptoms as fibromyalgia. These old texts spoke about autoimmune symptoms long before the diagnostic labels coming about. Here is how Ayurveda treats autoimmune symptoms:

1. Toxin removal: Ayurveda starts by working on removing the toxins from the body. According to Ayurveda, toxins or ama in the body interfere with the proper functioning of the immune system, which often leads to autoimmune diseases.

2. Metabolism correction: Ayurveda can correct the disordered metabolism evident in autoimmune conditions.

3. Increase in ojus production: Ojus is the component that helps in the nourishment of the immune system. It is generally received from the food you eat. Due to a dysfunctional immune system causing the impairment of metabolism, the production of ojus decreases. Ayurveda works to increases its production.

4. Immune system correction: Lastly, Ayurveda works to correct the immune system using various herbs to calm, correct and rejuvenate it.

137

Ayurveda looks at the autoimmune manifestation as an imbalance in the body doshas. When the body is brought into balance, the homeostatic balance results in the symptoms releasing. From my experience in Ayurvedic clinics, it is often a situation of too much vata and pitta.

For autoimmune treatment, it is likely that a long-term stay at an Ayurvedic clinic will be required (usually three weeks or more). I recommend looking at ones in India first as source is always best, but if that seems intimidating then Sri Lanka and Bali are close substitutes. There are two types of healing centres out there: ones designed for Ayurveda tourism and ones that are for a deeper healing process when a disease process has begun. If you need to test the waters, try a tourist version first. Ayurvedic centres can be strict and restrictive, with methods that may shock you. Please check in with your doctor whether this is appropriate for you at this time. Please also consult with the Ayurvedic doctors about what is happening with you before your visit so that they can tell you what they recommend in terms of length of time and whether their venue would be the most appropriate one for you. For women, try to avoid going during your menstrual cycle (if you are planning a short stay) as this may limit which treatments are accessible to you.

Colon hydrotherapy

Colon hydrotherapy is a good way to remove toxins in the gut and reduce inflammation in the gut lining. It is also known as colonic irrigation or colonic cleansing, and involves flushing the colon with fluids to remove waste. Colon hydrotherapy may have some risks and adverse side effects including mild cramping, abdominal pain, fullness, bloating, nausea, vomiting, dehydration, dizziness, electrolyte or mineral imbalance, bacterial imbalance, the potential to interfere with medication absorption on day of the procedure, bowel perforation, infection, depletion of normal bowel flora and kidney failure. It is contraindicated for those who have had colon surgery and people with heart or kidney disease, and it should be run past your doctor, especially if there are difficulties with the colon, such as Crohn's disease.

Colon hydrotherapy has been around since ancient times, and the benefits are based on the premise that digestive waste can be a toxin to the body – the body poisons itself by retaining waste. During a colon cleanse, large amounts of water – sometimes about 60 litres – and possibly other substances, such as herbs or coffee, are flushed through the colon using a tube inserted into the rectum. The practitioner then massages your abdomen and when you release the fluids, the waste is flushed from your colon.

It is useful for digestive issues such as bloating, colitis, constipation and indigestion, and non-digestive problems that include arthritis, allergies, chronic fatigue, asthma and skin conditions. When bodies are in good health, they are equipped to cleanse themselves – or to do so, perhaps, using simple aids like probiotics, exercise, hydration, good bowel routines and laxatives. The main theory behind colon cleansing is autointoxication – that undigested meat and other food builds up mucus in the colon, which produces toxins and feeds pathogens. Symptoms of this include fatigue, headaches, weight gain and low energy. Benefits of colon cleansing include improved mood, improved immune system, weight loss, improved clarity of skin, and reduced risk of colon cancer.

Ayurveda integrates colon hydrotherapy in the form of enemas (or basti) in its processes, often also delivering herbs and medications in this manner. This involves a gentle preparation of the body over a few days, in which a cleansing process is already in action. The western version of colon hydrotherapy often omits this preparation process, so it can sometimes feel like a shock or be harsh on the body. Please select your colon hydrotherapist carefully. Hygiene practices are of utmost importance here. Faecal material can move up the pipes, so these need to be replaced with every client. A good antiparasitic and probiotic may encourage the release of pathogens from your colon during this process. Probiotics should also be used during the process to replace and supplement good bacteria in the colon. The process is not comfortable, and you should feel that your symptoms are in a manageable phase if you choose to use this as a treatment.

BioScan

There are a few alternative methods that engage the power of technology in their methodology. One such method is called BioScan. The BioScan system is a testing machine that scans the body's organs and functions for imbalances using electrodermal screening. It is a procedure that combines the disciplines of acupuncture, biofeedback and homeopathy with laser light technology. It extracts the functional frequencies of your organs and systems by sending a current through the electrical pathways in the body (the meridians), providing a picture of whether you are functioning optimally or have chronic or acute blockages.

Every living thing has an electromagnetic field, blueprint and resonance. One of the basic principles of vibrational healing is that every part of the body, every cell, is in a state of vibration. When we are in a state of good health, our body has an overall harmonic output. However, when we encounter a frequency that is not harmonic, it causes disharmony that we then call dis-ease. Once the stressors are identified, your practitioner can quickly create a customised protocol to help this out-of-balance condition and put you on the path to an efficient and balanced state. This customised plan is a frequency generated by the machine and is then transmitted into you, and there may also be adjunct supplementation.

The machine can detect the presence of parasites, heavy metals, emotional trauma, physical body alignment problems, hormone dysregulation, allergies, problematic mitochondrial function and geopathic stress – faults in the ground, water, Wi-Fi/5G and radiation, among others.

Other machines like this exist – the SCIO is another well-known option. The principles of these machines are the same as ancient medicine systems – using frequency (or energy) to reharmonise the body.

Shamanic medicines

This level of assistance is perhaps for those who are a bit more open-minded to such things and it may not resonate with everyone reading this book. This route is something you must be ready for and there needs to be an intuitive calling for it. I will focus on two medicines in my discussion here – a psychedelic plant medicine called ayahuasca and Kambo, a secretion from the monkey frog (or leaf frog).

Certain plant-based psychedelics may have the ability to treat mental health difficulties, according to recent research. Modern psychiatry is beginning to consider the possibility of using substances such as psilocybin (magic mushrooms) for treating diagnoses such as depression and trauma. There is some research supporting the treatment of autoimmune conditions. Psychedelics may directly and indirectly target several physiological factors and resulting dysfunctions in autoimmune conditions via a number of different mechanisms. Biochemical and anecdotal evidence suggests that ayahuasca could provide a novel treatment approach to autoimmune and other immune and inflammation-related diseases.

Ayahuasca is specifically under investigation due to its combination of effects that may affect autoimmunity. Ayahuasca is a psychedelic substance originating in the Amazon that is used for healing, personal development and religious purposes. Evidence shows that it has anti-inflammatory and immune-modulating effects. One human study where ayahuasca was given to healthy volunteers recorded blood levels of lymphocytes and found a decrease in CD4 and CD3 cells, and an increase in NK cells. The therapeutic outcome of psychedelic-assisted psychotherapy could resolve or improve stressful psychological states that cause or contribute to the physiological outcomes seen in most autoimmune patients. Ayahuasca could be a pathway to working with deeply repressed and intergenerational trauma in your DNA – often things that psychotherapy may struggle to access adequately.

As you've seen, chronic low-grade infections of bacteria, fungi and viruses are rife in autoimmune conditions. There is evidence to suggest that psychedelic compounds, such as ayahuasca, may have an antimicrobial activity against these organisms. Antifungal properties have been demonstrated, as well as an antiviral action against herpes simplex 2, which is common in autoimmune conditions. It may be that through its action on trauma through the HPA axis, a biochemical cascade could result in ayahuasca helping to re-regulate the gut microbiome. Additionally, the longevity, physical vigour and mental acuity evidenced by many ayahuasca shamans in Peru has long been noted as remarkable. Many of these shamans living in developing nations are well into their seventies, eighties and nineties, yet appear to live out their years in a state of physical and mental health that would be the envy of many in the so-called developed countries. Certainly, some of this is due to dietary factors and a physically vigorous and demanding lifestyle; but some of it may be the result of exceptional immune functions due to their years of working with ayahuasca. Many of these practitioners are accustomed to consuming it several times a week in the performance of their healing practices and have done so for most of their adult lives.

When it comes to autoimmunity and ayahuasca, the chemistry in your body is already in chaos. Ayahuasca is going to send your brain chemistry into chaos. Make sure you are ready. Integrating the insights that ayahuasca delivers is hard work – you need to have capacity and space to be able to do that. When you are already feeling dysregulated emotionally and have lots of body symptoms, adding the anxiety, adrenaline and intensity of an ayahuasca journey may not be the right path. Ayahuasca involves purging, shaking, crying and much physical expression through the body. If your body is fragile, you may not want to put yourself through this. There is evidence that ayahuasca has antiparasitic qualities, so it may help you rid yourself of the pathogens inside you. On the other hand, there is evidence that ayahuasca may lower the immune system's effectiveness for a few days after use – if you are in the midst of some sort of acute infection, perhaps it is worth waiting until that settles.

Other research has showed that ayahuasca seems to affect how we cope with a disease in a positive way. Coping includes all kinds of aspects of handling a disease: acceptance, a positive way of life, relaxation, and so on. In addition, there is a tendency for people to use ayahuasca before an illness manifests itself in the body, for preventive purposes. Participants insist on the idea that before problems manifest in the 'material dimension', they exist in the 'spiritual dimension'. Ayahuasca is a medium for working in these dimensions. By ingesting ayahuasca, you can reach an emotional–spiritual dimension in which the 'true' cause of an illness can be discovered and influenced, and the body's self-healing can be activated.

One study has listed some profound ayahuasca-related changes that may be useful for chronic illness:

1. A change in health behaviours, including diet, and abstaining from alcohol or cigarettes
2. Enhanced clarity, recognition and sensibility
3. Increased physical well-being
4. Energy, power and strength
5. Greater ability to cope with problems and daily hassles
6. Confidence and tranquillity
7. A renewed sense of happiness, love and joy
8. A change of life orientation, sometimes including striving for non-materialistic values
9. Improved social competencies, including emotions like gratitude, forgiveness and humility.

All participants expressed the idea that ayahuasca helped them by activating or stimulating their self-healing powers. This idea is often connected with the concept of an 'inner healer'. This is based on the belief that everybody has the wisdom and the power to heal any illness without the need of invasive procedures or pharmaceutical drugs. People who have this idea do not consider themselves passive patients, but active contributors to their healing process.

Indigenous people in the Amazon have used Kambo, an excretion from a frog, for centuries to heal and cleanse the body by strengthening its natural defences and warding off bad luck. It is also believed to increase stamina and hunting skills. Kambo is believed to assist with addictions, anxiety, cancer, chronic pain, depression, diabetes, infections, rheumatism, HIV and Alzheimer's disease. Certain types of peptides found in Kambo have powerful antimicrobial properties, so it fights drug-resistant strains of bacteria, yeast, parasites and viruses.

Kambo use entails burning the skin and placing the excretions of the monkey frog into these burns. A reaction happens where vomiting, or purging, is induced. Unlike ayahuasca, Kambo has no mind-altering qualities. It is believed that Kambo can heal autoimmune conditions, but research is yet to investigate this.

Please err on the side of caution when using these methods. Ayahuasca can be an intensive process in which retraumatisation is not impossible. Ayahuasca may do in one session what psychotherapy does in years, but are we ready to confront all this in one sitting? What is the rush? I have found in my practice that people who use ayahuasca frequently have no defences. They tend to sometimes become very sensitive, overempathetic and easily triggered, and sometimes develop magical ideas that alienate them from their family, friendships or community. Those who have used ayahuasca from a traumatised state often have an overstimulated HPA axis – they are stuck on 'on' – and sometimes this entails replaying the trauma memories that they have processed over and over, which becomes a trauma in itself. The newfound way of 'seeing' that ayahuasca brings may create difficulties with going back to life as it was before – and perhaps the foundations for escaping that life have not been set up yet. Kambo has been known to overstimulate the immune system and cause an unwanted response, so it is not all clear-cut. I know desperate times call for desperate measures, but do your research, consult your doctor and perhaps a psychiatrist, and choose wisely.

Personal healing practices

There are some solutions that are within your control. The body needs to be cleansed and supported with adequate nutrition and hydration. Your adrenals need to be calmed through various strategies. Your self-healing powers and resilience need activation. Connection in your life needs to be re-established – to people, to nature and to your own self. This section discusses the areas in which you can begin to take control.

Repairing the body

You should have three goals for your body: repairing deficient organ function, reducing inflammation, and detoxification.

Repairing organ function

Fatty liver

There are many liver-cleansing systems and diets, but the best one seems to involve a lot of raw foods focusing on lemon, kale, parsley and spinach, and avoiding alcohol, added sugar, deep-fried foods, added salt, white bread, rice, pasta and red meat. The liver likes bitter and calciferous vegetables. Supplements that assist the liver include vitamin B2, choline and glutathione. Coconut oil helps the liver. Milk thistle is the best herb for healing the liver.

What worked for me was the *Medical Medium* book I mentioned earlier. It is a controversial book in the medical community in terms of its claims about autoimmune diseases, and it may not be up everyone's alley that there are psychic aspects involved in obtaining this information, but the action and the effectiveness of the diet that Coviello puts forward in that book cannot be denied. Many swear by the positive effects it has had for them. On the *Medical Medium* detox, I would have a smoothie with the following for breakfast daily: blueberries, banana, apple, raspberries, walnuts or pecan nuts, papaya or melon, spinach, coriander, spirulina powder, barley grass powder, pitaya (dragon fruit) powder, Atlantic dulse, cat's claw, fresh orange juice and ashwagandha. I would also drink some celery juice and hot lemon ginger tea in the morning. Lunch would be a raw soup with tomato, orange, spinach, garlic and basil. Dinner would be a salad of kale, bean sprouts, apple, papaya, walnuts or pecan nuts and dried cranberries with a lemon, honey and orange juice dressing. I would have some ostrich, grilled fish, butternut soup and potato here and there when I needed something warm to eat.

Leaky gut

A healthy gut allows nutrients to be absorbed and blocks the absorption of toxins and pathogens. Most women, unfortunately, do not empty their bowels adequately when going to the toilet. It is as though in the female psychology, a quick and small poo is all that is allowed for us to maintain our femininity. Most men are known for taking their newspaper (now their cellphone) to the toilet and having a good sit on the loo. The first place to start healing your gut is perhaps your toilet habits.

To heal the gut, we need to remove the most common reactive foods and replenish digestive enzymes. In some cases, enzymes can also help remove infections by 'digesting' the infectious organism or breaking down its protein-containing hiding spot. Simultaneously, we need to supply the body with the nutrients it needs to heal, and we must re-establish balance in our gut flora by encouraging pathogenic bacteria to leave peacefully while replenishing beneficial bacteria. We can summarise this as follows:

1. Remove (gluten, dairy, grains, bad oils, sugar, raw vegetables, egg white, cold drinks)
2. Reseal (bone broth, sprouted rice, cooked veggies, pumpkin, pears, blueberries and herbs)
3. Reseed (probiotics)
4. Rebuild (bone broth, ginger, astragalus, collagen and zinc)
5. Restore (manage your emotions as your gut is your second brain).

Adrenal fatigue

Body stress must be extracted. Somatic psychotherapy, yoga and trauma release exercises should be the first port of call here. Some nutritional things you can do include taking vitamin B1, potassium and magnesium. Herbs such as valerian and chamomile may assist. These will help support the nervous system and calm the body. Sleep, especially REM sleep, will assist in regulating the body out of traumatised states. Low-intensity exercise is important, especially walking, and lots of breathing to pull the stress out of the body.

Address inflammation

Anti-inflammatory herbs and supplements include turmeric (or curcumin, which is the bioactive substance in turmeric that works on inflammation), ginger, vitamin D3, MSM, arnica and omega-3 fatty acids. Omega-3 does not agree with everybody as a healing supplement, and there is some evidence that some forms of this may contain mercury. A useful method of lowering inflammation in your body is to move to a raw fruit and vegetable diet for some time. This is not only alkalising, but also detoxing. Other aspects to consider that may reduce inflammation include safe social connection, gentle exercise, stimulating playful experiences, oxygen, an alkaline diet, sleep, massage and stress reduction.

Detoxification

You need to cleanse to heal. If your body is burdened with toxins, it cannot heal. However, strong detoxes too early may further impair your gut and adrenals, as well as deprive you of the nutrients of a complete diet. First support the body and heal the detox organs and pathways in your body so that your body is able to release what you cleanse from your system. Start by removing all triggering foods from your diet and then add supportive foods. Increase your intake of raw foods. If this doesn't work for you, I recommend trying puréed or softened warm foods, as Ayurveda uses in its detoxes. This is a gentler approach and may increase the absorption of nutrients.

The best way to cleanse your body is through diet (including increasing your intake of fibre and antioxidant foods, and reducing salt, added sugar and processed foods), juicing, colon cleanses, salt baths, massages, using steaming or saunas, exercise and hydration. Limiting exposure to toxins is a key first step. Detoxing involves creating the right environment in your body so that your organs can more efficiently do what they do naturally. Your body can get rid of toxins on its own if you bring about these conditions. When we have an autoimmune condition, we are more sensitive to these toxins and hold on to them a lot more. Detox pathways in some bodies may also cease to work – many autoimmune patients in my practice, for example, no longer sweat. Part of improving organ function is to reduce inflammation in the body.

It is best to do detoxes and fasts under supervision until you know what you are doing. During any detoxification process, it is important to note that your body will pass through a healing crisis in which it can often feel worse, with symptoms such as fatigue, headaches, fogginess or altered digestion. You may experience numerous healing crises on your healing journey as various pathogens die off, heavy metals are released, or toxins are cleared. These are the body's responses to ridding itself of toxic elements and will only last for as long as the body needs to let go of what it is releasing. Don't confuse this healing crisis with illness. Fasting can also be a form of detoxing (more about this later). You may need to add heavy metal cleanses into the mix at a later stage – but note that these can be hard on the body, so perhaps do the detoxing in layers. Chlorella, spirulina and zeolite powder are useful for clearing heavy metals out of the body. Check zeolite powders for the presence of aluminium, as this may be counterproductive. Be aware that doing a heavy metal cleanse when the heavy metal source (such as an amalgam filling) is still present in your body may lead to flare-ups. It is recommended that you remove the source of the heavy metal first, or that you do the cleanse under the guidance of an experienced practitioner.

For me, the most important part of cleansing is drinking vegetable juices. Overdoing detoxing and juicing may, however, be another way of overstimulating the adrenal system, so again, move into this gradually.

Once your body is clean, you can more clearly assess other aspects of your life. Detoxification can then be extended to all areas of life. You can detox your home from excess clutter, your relationships from those that are not good for you, and your diary from activities that don't add value to you.

The next natural place to go to is diet, as this is one of the methods you will use to detoxify.

Diet

Due to the influence of pathogens, toxins and trauma, your body is not functioning inside as it should. So, it needs the greatest support you can offer in terms of lifestyle and diet. Your body is not absorbing nutrients adequately due to decreased organ function. It also requires increased nutrition as it is fighting pathogens.

Food is medicine. The food you eat contains everything your body needs to heal, as long as you are eating the right things. As mentioned earlier, the problem with our food today is that some of the soils in which is it grown lack an effective microbiome, making it nutrient deficient. We are fed by a food industry that pays no attention to health, and treated by a health industry that pays no attention to food. Consider that, right now, every bite you take needs to maximise the delivery of nutrition to the body.

One of the first steps you can take is to begin to eat only whole foods – foods that are as close to their natural, unprocessed form as possible. Do not eat anything manufactured. I have discussed some important dietary aspects below, but this deserves a book in itself. Getting your diet right is an integral part of this journey. How you eat also needs to be considered. Our fast-paced lifestyles often result in fast-paced eating. It's time to become mindful of each bite.

The Autoimmune Protocol Diet

The best way to eat is perhaps to look back at our ancestors. This likely looks like a paleo diet, which has a high level of alkaline food content. Our ancestors likely didn't eat meat daily. They probably didn't eat seeds, as they would plant these. Processed food didn't exist, and the practice of using animal dairy may not have been established yet.

The Autoimmune Protocol Diet (AIP) is a food-based approach to eliminating unwanted inflammation from the body. It is thought to help heal your gut, reduce inflammation created by autoimmune conditions. It is equated to the paleo diet, at least in its initial stages.

It begins with an elimination phase, in which you remove everything that may be driving the problems in your body. In the elimination phase, foods and medication that are believed to cause gut inflammation, imbalances between levels of good and bad bacteria, or an immune response are removed – foods like grains, legumes, nuts, nightshade vegetables (tomatoes, eggplant, potatoes and peppers), eggs and dairy are completely removed. This helps you localise food sensitivities and the food that is making you unwell. Tobacco, alcohol, coffee, oil, food additives, refined and processed sugars, and anti-inflammatory medications should be avoided. This phase encourages the consumption of fresh, nutrient-dense foods, minimally processed, organic free-range meat, fermented foods and bone broth. It focuses on meat, vegetables and fruit. It also speaks to improving lifestyle factors simultaneously: stress, sleep and physical activity. The elimination phase is maintained until the individual experiences a noticeable reduction in symptoms. As a guideline, this is usually 30–90 days. Most people notice improvements within the initial weeks.

The next phase is the reintroduction phase, in which foods you have been avoiding are gradually reintroduced into the diet, one at a time, based on your tolerance. The goal here is to identify which foods contribute to your symptoms and to reintroduce all foods that don't cause symptoms, while continuing to avoid the ones that do, to allow for the widest dietary variety you can tolerate. You allow about a week to pass between reintroducing different foods. This way, you can notice any reappearing symptoms before any further reintroductions. Once you have added a food back into your diet and have stayed symptom free, that food can stay in your diet.

It is best not to test foods like gluten, and to leave them out of your diet permanently. Many people prefer to stay on the classic paleo diet as they enjoy being symptom free and the weight control benefit this diet offers. This diet is simple to follow, and as long as the intake of fruit and vegetables exceeds that of meat, it likely offers the best diet management solution for autoimmune conditions. There are, however, some diets suggested for autoimmune conditions that promote higher intakes of meat, fish and eggs as a start, such as the GAPS diet ('gut and psychology syndrome'). This diet restricts all grains, commercial dairy, starchy foods and all processed and refined carbohydrates, and encourages easily digestible and nutrient-dense foods. However, it also believes in reducing foods that may be harsh on the gut lining (raw/excessive plant food). Most of the foods on the GAPS diet consist of meat, fish, eggs, fermented foods, homemade dairy and well-cooked vegetables. Gradually as symptoms subside, foods are added to re-establish a complete diet.

This diet supports the phase in healing where the body needs to be re-established, but perhaps does not support detoxification, and perhaps it sets up conditions where some pathogens may flourish under high acidity in the body. It does, however, deliver a higher number of amino acids which allow the body to rebuild itself.

The acid–alkaline diet

The acid–alkaline diet theory is one I always keep at the back of my mind when balancing my food intake daily. The theory, although disputed by many, is that you can alter the pH value of your body through your diet and thus create a particular environment in your body.

Your metabolism (the conversion of food to energy) is compared to fire (agni) in Ayurvedic traditions. When your metabolism breaks down the foods you eat, an 'ash' is left as a residue. This metabolic waste can be alkaline, neutral or acidic. Acidic bodies are believed to be more vulnerable to illness, whereas alkaline environments are protective or resistant to this. 'Acidic' means pH values of between 0 and 6,9. 'Neutral' means a pH of 7. And 'alkaline' means pH values of between 7,1 and 14. Diabetes, starvation or alcohol intake can cause pH levels to fall into an acidic state. This is difficult to verify scientifically as different parts of the body have different pH states. For example, it is normal for the stomach to be highly acidic due to the presence of hydrochloric acid that is used to digest food.

Your blood needs to stay at a constant pH level for you to remain healthy. Generally, a healthy body is able to manage its own pH levels, but an autoimmune body may struggle here due to toxin and pathogen overload, needing some external support.

Following a diet based on the pH levels of different foods seems to alleviate most people's difficulties with persistent infections. Medical science offers limited treatment for viruses (antivirals, even, only work in specific window periods) and this diet may help you solve this problem. Most bacteria, viruses and fungi don't thrive when you are consuming an alkaline diet, but you need to have eaten this way for a long time to achieve this. Foods that are cited as being 'acid producing' include meat, wheat and other grains, refined sugar, dairy, caffeine and alcohol. Stress is also cited as shifting the body into an acidic state. Foods that are considered alkaline are fruits and vegetables. Many believe that, to maintain a constant pH level in your blood, your body takes alkaline minerals such as

pH Chart

		High Alkaline Ionised Water		
Consume Freely Raw is Best	**10**	Raw Spinach Brussels Sprouts Cauliflower Alfafa Grass Seaweeds	Raw Brocolli Red Cabbage Carrots Cucumbers Asparagus	Artichokes Raw Celery Potato Skins Collards Lemons & Limes
Alkaline pH	**9.0**	Olive Oil Raw Zucchini Sprouted Grains Raw Green beans Mangoes Tangerines Grapes	Most Lettuce Sweet Potato Raw Egg Plant Blueberries Papayas Melons	Borage Oil Raw Peas Alfafa Sprouts Pears Figs & Dates Kiwi
Most foods get more acidic when cooked	**8.0**	Apples Tomatoes Turnip Bell peppers Pineapple Wild Rice Canteloupe Oranges	Almonds Fresh Corn Olives Radish Cherries Strawberries Honeydew Grapefruit	Avocaos Mushrooms Soybeans Rhubarb Millet Apricots Peaches Bananas
	7.0	**MOST TAP WATER** Municipalities adjust tap water to be ± 7.0 Optimum pH for HUMAN BLODD is 7.365		Butter, fresh, unsalt Cream, fresh, raw Milk, Raw cow's Margarine Oils, except Olive
It take 30 parts of ALKALINITY to neutralise 1 part ACIDITY in the body	**6.0**	Milk, Yoghurt Most Grains Eggs Kidney Beans Processed Juices Brown Rice Sprouted Wheat Bread Oysters	Fruit Juices Soy Milk, Goat's Milk Fish Lima Beans Rye Bread Cocoa Oats Cold Water Fish	Cooked Spinach Coconut Tea Plums Spelt Rice & Almond Milk Liver Salmon, Tuna
	5.0	Cooked Beans Sugar Potatoes w/o Skins Garbanzos Butter, salted WHeat Bran	Chicken & Turkey Canned FruitPinto Beans Lentils Rice Cakes Rhubarb Beer	White Rice Navy Beans Black Beans Cooked Corn Molassses
Alkaline pH **Consume sparingly or never**	**4.0**	Reverse Osmosis Water Coffee Pistachios Cranberries Wheat Popcorn	Distilled & Purified Water White Bread Beef Prunes Most Nuts	Peanuts **Most Bottled Water & Sports Drinks** Blackberries Sweetened Fruit Juices Tomato Sauce
	3.0	Lamb Shellfish Goat Cheeese Pasta Worry Tobacco Smoke Sweet'N Low Nutrasweet	Posrk pastries soda Pickles Lack of Sleep Chocolate Equal Process Food	Wine Cheese Black Tea Stress Overwork Vinegar Aspartame Microwaved Foods

2.3 Colas! (Off the Chart)

calcium from your bones to buffer the acids from the acid-forming foods you eat. This may cause a loss in bone mineral density that could be linked to osteoporosis. Most theories, however, don't support this, and protein may actually be beneficial for bones.

There is no doubt that those who eat more of an acid (or keto) diet are more prone to infections such as flu – if you are prone to more minor infections, then you are certainly prone to more major ones. So, even though this thinking is controversial, it is worth considering pH levels in your choices of food. Proponents say that your diet should consist of 75 per cent of alkaline foods, and 25 per cent of acidic foods. Look at the chart that follows for guidance.

I believe that this form of eating can be integrated into the AIP diet and that, together, they should guide how you eat.

No to keto

The ketogenic diet can be quite extreme for people with autoimmune disease. I don't recommend this diet when you are in a place of healing. There have, however, been some studies that show that this diet has a positive effect on epilepsy and diabetes, as well as heart disease, cancer (it may slow tumour growth), Alzheimer's disease, Parkinson's disease and PCOS. If you have these conditions and you choose to attempt this diet, please do so under strict guidance of a practitioner who specialises in this. It is preferable to make this diet a temporary intervention.

The aim of the keto diet is to force your body into using fuel that comes from fat rather than from glucose. You then use the stored fat in your body, which helps you lose weight. Most of the healthy individuals I have seen attempt this diet lost a lot of weight in a short space of time, but it seemed like a stormy experience due to the 'keto flu' they experienced and symptoms such as diarrhoea, constipation, vomiting, poor energy and mental function, increased hunger, sleep issues, nausea, digestive discomfort, and decreased exercise performance. These symptoms may be unbearable on top of a list of autoimmune symptoms.

This diet puts excessive strain on the liver through the extra fat the liver needs to process. If you have a virus in your system that is already weighing down your liver, any extra pressure may exacerbate your current condition instead of improving it. If you have any pathogens or parasites, they are going to have a party with what is going to be going on inside your liver with all the additional fat. Your detoxification pathways are also going to be blocked. Other risks include a low level of protein in the blood, kidney stones and micronutrient deficiencies.

A ketogenic diet may also change the water and mineral balance in your body, so it may be necessary to take a mineral supplement. Another difficulty is that this diet can give you permission to eat unhealthily. Most of this diet should focus on foods such as meat, fish, eggs, butter, nuts, healthy oils, avocados and low-carb vegetables. But many end up eating fried breakfasts, an abundance of pork and other foods that are far away from anything healing. Many people who go on this diet also experience increased acidity in their bodies, which makes them more prone to illness. This is not ideal for someone with an already vulnerable immune system.

Vegetarian and vegan diets

Vegetarian and vegan diets have become more popular in recent years for reasons of personal health and animal treatment. Vegetarianism has become aligned with consciousness. Vegetarian and vegan diets require much effort to ensure that adequate protein, B vitamins and iron are delivered to the body. They may result in a vitamin B_{12} deficiency, so please check this and supplement if required.

Also worth checking are your iron levels. Iron is available in a vegetarian diet, but it does require eating foods that aren't popular with the palate. Please check your levels regularly if you choose this type of diet and have an autoimmune condition. Certain plants, seeds and nuts have pro-inflammatory associations, and nuts like cashews have a naturally occurring mould that may make healing bodies flare up. Vegan processed food may not be good for you, as it is often infused with soya and gluten as protein substitutes. There is something to be said for eating natural, unprocessed, whole foods, as nature intended.

A diet high in fruit and vegetables creates a dominantly alkaline environment in the body, in which pathogens cannot survive. If eradicating pathogens is your aim, this kind of diet will certainly do the trick. But if there is damage to the body, the nutrients from meat products may indeed be required. If you consider how much plant material a cow, for example, consumes, and the energetic frequency in its body as a consequence of this consumption, it may make sense at times in the healing process to consume this concentrated energy. Eating various meat products may also assist in balancing certain hormones, which are frequently out of balance in autoimmune conditions.

Fasting

Fasting and the latest intermittent fasting trend are alternative health approaches that have cleansing and healing properties. Unfortunately, these are very stressful on the adrenals. Intermittent fasting is a term used for meal timing schedules that cycle between voluntary fasting and non-fasting over a given period. It is more focused on when you should eat than on what you should eat.

When you fast, certain things happen in your cells and hormones. Firstly, your body adjusts hormone levels to make stored body fat more accessible. Human growth hormone (HGH) levels increase, which benefits repair and muscle gain. Your cells initiate repair processes as they are not occupied with the process of digestion and nutrient absorption. When you are healing, your body may benefit more from reducing the size of meals than eliminating them. Your autoimmune condition has affected your body's ability to absorb nutrients, so removing regular nutrition can cause discomfort such as anxiety, restlessness or pain.

You can use fasting when your body feels burdened by flu or a stomach bug to take the pressure off the digestive system so that the body can focus on fighting the virus. Instead of fasting, perhaps focus on eating smaller meals, which keeps the blood sugar stable. A recommendation for when you are healing: have dinner at 4 p.m. at the latest so that your body experiences a gentle, intermittent fast overnight, when it can focus on detoxing and rebuilding rather than on digestion. Once your body is in a more regulated, detoxed space, you can consider fasting, preferably later in the healing journey. I have seen much psychological benefit to fasting in that it forces you to be with what is going on inside you, without using food as a means of coping and to distract you from your emotions.

Cooking your food

Ayurveda believes that for illness it is best to consume warm, cooked foods, as these put less stress on the digestive system and are gentler on the body. For a body that is very unwell, it could be a good place to begin with puréed and warm food – vegetable soups, for example. Some foods contain dangerous bacteria and microorganisms that are only eliminated by cooking, and avoiding further infection is important when healing.

Cooking foods is believed to deactivate the enzymes found in them. However, there is no evidence that food enzymes contribute to better health. Some nutrients are easily deactivated or can leach out of food during the cooking process, while others become more available for your body to use. Water-soluble vitamins, such as vitamin C and the B vitamins, are particularly susceptible to being lost during cooking. It is likely that some foods are better raw, and others are better cooked. Cooking breaks down plants' fibres and cell walls, which better prepares some of the nutrients within the cells to be absorbed. This is important when digestion requires support for the absorption of nutrients. Eat a combination of cooked and raw foods for maximum health benefits.

With various cooking methods available, your aim should be to retain a high number of the food's nutrients. Steaming, roasting and stir-frying are some of the best methods of cooking vegetables when it comes to retaining nutrients. Boiling results in a loss of nutritional content. Deep frying, smoking and grilling often form carcinogens. Air frying is a good alternative to frying. There is some research evidence to indicate that continuous ingestion of microwaved food may cause immune system deficiencies through lymph gland and blood serum alteration. When frying foods, consider the oils you may be using. Canola, corn, cottonseed, sunflower, safflower, soy, grapeseed, palm, wheat germ, peanut and rice bran oils are industrial oils that should be avoided. These become especially toxic to the body when heated. Margarine, most vegan butters and other butter substitutes should be avoided too. The winner when it comes to high-heat cooking is coconut oil. Over 90 per cent of the fatty acids in it are saturated, which makes it very resistant to heat. A close second is avocado oil. Olive oil is a healthy oil but cannot handle temperatures that are as high. Ghee and butter are good at high temperatures and nutritious, as long as they are sourced from the right places (more about this later).

Eating for organs

There is a theory that the food you need to heal a particular organ looks like that organ. It can be considered that everything around us has some sort of intelligent design, and there are definite patterns in life, so perhaps this theory is correct.

We can start with the walnut, which – with its many folds and wrinkles – looks quite similar to the brain. Walnuts have a high concentration of omega-3 fatty acids, which are indeed good for brain health. These fatty acids are extremely helpful in protecting brain health and improving cognitive performance.

A bunch of celery stalks can be said to resemble bones. Celery contains about 23 per cent sodium, which is a similar composition to that of our bones. Celery seeds have a high calcium and manganese content that helps increase bone mineral density and bone structure for longer, healthier bones.

Sweet potatoes can be said to resemble the pancreas. The pancreas is responsible for breaking down food from the stomach and producing insulin to help balance the body's glucose levels. Sweet potatoes can help adjust the glycaemic index, which can aid pancreatic function.

And ginger resembles the stomach. It is known to aid in digestion and various stomach ailments, including nausea and morning sickness.

Eating for symptoms

Eating for symptoms is another way to look your diet. If you have a virus in your system, eating lots of antiviral foods will assist you. Eating onions, garlic and ginger, and drinking coconut water, will help you fight the virus in your system. Onions and garlic are stimulants and excellent prebiotics. They also have strong antimicrobial (antiviral and antibacterial) properties. Chicken broth is rich in collagen and may be good for joint pain and gut healing, but it is highly acidic – in some people, it could exacerbate joint pain. Ginger may assist you with nausea. Nuts, fatty fish, leafy greens (and of course hydration!) are good for headaches and migraines.

The *Medical Medium* books have gained popularity in promoting a diet aimed at eliminating EBV. This diet focuses on integrating specific fruit and vegetables into your repertoire, as they have certain functions or treat certain symptoms in the body. According to this diet, blueberries are believed to remove neurotoxins from the liver – they have the highest antioxidant content of any fruit or vegetable. Celery strengthens the immune and reproductive systems. Bananas heal the nerves attached to the digestive tract. Spinach rebuilds digestive health. Kale helps protect the lungs. Atlantic dulse supports the thyroid. Spirulina helps rebuild the CNS. Barley grass removes toxins and other heavy metals from the blood. Apples prevent dehydration, stave off bacteria, yeast and mould from the gut, and help the body recover from stress. Melon hydrates skin, nails and the nervous system. Oranges remove toxins from of the digestive tract, help sinus and respiratory issues, and cleanse the gallbladder. Lemon improves hydrochloric acid production in the stomach. Pomegranates support healthy blood flow and clean blood vessels. Cherries strengthen the circulatory system. Cranberries prevent oxidation of cells. Potatoes help fight viruses in body. Asparagus has powerful anti-inflammatory properties. Coriander cleanses and strengthens the liver and removes heavy metals from the body – it is a natural chelator. Broccoli supports the immune system, and helps fight bacteria and other bugs in the intestinal tract. Pears support the adrenals. Onions are a powerful antiviral. Papayas reduce gut inflammation.

Fruit

Fruit is important to healing, so if you do have difficulties with sugar, please check with your doctor whether it would be possible to incorporate some lower-sugar fruits into your diet. I understand that in diabetes this needs to be limited, but some of the diabetics I have seen in my practice swear that fruit does not have a negative effect on their sugar. I am not sure why this is, but if there is a window that allows you to eat fruit, then do it! It has a bad reputation due to its sugar content but remember, this is a good sugar. Fruit is also very satisfying to eat – it creates vitality in our systems. Some eastern traditions believe that eating fruit is linked to higher levels of consciousness.

Eating for PTSD

Since PTSD is a big driver of autoimmune conditions, consider eating in a way that ameliorates PTSD. In Ayurveda, PTSD points to imbalanced vata and pitta, with both being too high. So, foods that may ameliorate PTSD include vata- and pitta-pacifying foods. I recommend eating warm, sweet foods (natural sugars from fruit and vegetables, not artificial sugar), with spices such as nutmeg, cardamon and cinnamon to balance the energies. Foods that stabilise the adrenals and regular meals may help to regulate adrenaline levels, as may gluten-free grains such as millet. Blueberries are believed to be a PTSD-healing food.

Prebiotic and probiotic foods

Foods that contain prebiotics and probiotics are very important to support your immune system and repopulate the gut and body with the right type of bacteria. Prebiotic foods include onions and garlic. Fermented foods are filled with probiotics that support gut and detoxification pathways. These include kefir, kombucha, sauerkraut, pickles, miso, tempeh, nattō and kimchi. Fermented coconut yoghurt, fermented coconut water and fermented cabbage are a few of my favourites.

Some of these may be worth debating health-wise, like kombucha, which can contain added sugars and is made on a black tea base. Yoghurt may not be an ideal source of probiotics since dairy blocks the body's detoxification pathways.

The bacteria found in fermented foods can be beneficial in balancing your intestinal flora and can help with constipation, digestion and anxiety. If you buy fermented foods, including cabbage, be sure to pick the kinds that are kept in the fridge. Probiotic bacteria can only survive for a couple of weeks at room temperature.

Source your food from the right places

If you eat meat, you need to look at the quality of the meat you are consuming. Never consume animals that have been treated badly or are in the mass production system – you are consuming trauma energetically. This dysregulates your ANS, flaring up your adrenals.

Farming practices have been modified to provide for mass production of animal produce to feed an ever-increasing global population. This includes practices such as force-feeding chickens using pipes down their throats so that they grow faster. Various kinds of hormones are given to cows to stimulate milk production, and to chicken to stimulate growth, among other things. You then consume these hormones, which wreak havoc on your own hormones.

Pesticides in plants are no better. Growing technologies have increased the amount of chemicals that are put into soil so that crops can be grown in record time. Soils are over-farmed, and the microbiome of the earth is not adequately restored. Rainwater contains chemicals, not the minerals it once did. Consider the sources of your food.

Foods to avoid

There are foods you should avoid when healing. Gluten deserves a section all of its own. Gluten-free diets have become very popular due to an awareness of the health complications from gluten consumption. Gluten is common in food such as pizza, pasta and cereal. It is frequently added to processed foods to improve texture and promote water retention. So, check those vegan sausages if you eat that sort of thing! It sneaks itself into food in restaurants – for example, flour is used to thicken vegetable soups, so be on the lookout for this.

Gluten is protein found in many grains, including wheat, barley, and rye. Most grains have it, so it is probably easier to list the ones that don't: brown rice, sorghum, quinoa, buckwheat, amaranth, millet and teff. Millet is a good grain to eat in that it is also alkaline. Oats are a difficult one: they don't typically contain gluten but are processed in environments that have been contaminated with gluten.

Gluten provides no essential nutrients. It is a problem for almost everyone with autoimmune conditions due to underlying intestinal issues, sensitivity to allergens and intolerance to anything that may cause increased inflammation. Gluten difficulty may manifest in various ways such as digestive issues (diarrhoea, bloating, abdominal pain, constipation, inflammation of digestive tissues), skin problems (rashes, eczema and skin inflammation), neurological issues (confusion, fatigue, anxiety, numbness, depression, lack of focus and difficulty speaking), weight loss or gain, nutrient deficiencies, diminished immune function, osteoporosis, anaemia and headaches.

As a start I would eliminate all soya, dairy, corn, legumes, eggs, farmed fish, seeds, seed oils, added sugars, anything processed, anything from a can, all grains (including gluten), and meat that contains hormones, to give your body the best possible conditions for finding its balance again. Soya has an impact on the endocrine system through increasing oestrogen levels, and excess oestrogen is common in people with autoimmunity. As you've seen, dairy can block the body's detoxification pathways, causing mucus build-up. Seeds and seed oils may be pro-inflammatory. Corn often gets contaminated by fungi that produce mycotoxins, which slow down the immune system. It is also often genetically modified.

Nature creates a perfect design – it creates food that, when ingested, heals and vibrates our energy system in a way that restores our flow and vitality. Stay away from the unnatural – that food will not be your medicine. Get in touch with your intuition and listen to what your body needs from day to day, and notice how this may change. Monitor your skin, your eyes, your hair, your tongue, your bowel movements and especially your symptoms, and learn what makes you better.

I am almost guaranteed a flare-up if I eat gluten. So, what do you do if you have eaten something that flares you up? Try these:

- Hot lemon water
- Epsom salts bath (to draw out the toxins)
- Activated charcoal
- Aloe tablets (if you can tolerate this, to help expel the substance sooner)
- Green juice (celery, spinach, kale and cucumber) in abundance
- Quercetin and vitamin C
- Lemon balm tea.

Hydration

Many of us are chronically dehydrated. Most of the fluids we consume daily, such as coffee, alcohol and sodas, actually dehydrate us. It is also important to consider the dehydrating effects of toxins and pathogens on the body.

Dehydration creates conditions for pathogens to thrive, so there is a feedback loop here: the more dehydrated you are, the greater your viral load, and the more dehydrated you become. Viruses can sometimes thicken or clot the blood. Hydration can help reduce the thickness of the blood so it can flow more easily through the system, oxygenating your system adequately. The more oxygen in your body, the greater your healing.

Another factor to consider in hydration is your salt intake. The salt volumes in restaurant and packaged food are often too high and can be detrimental to the functioning of your body. Adequate sodium levels are important, but this is better sourced from foods such as celery and spinach than from refined salt. You may need to lower your salt intake to assist hydration.

Hydration is important for detoxification. If you are properly hydrated, your body can remove toxins from the liver and kidneys effectively. Lemon juice in hot water is a good way to start the day, to activate the liver and provide hydration. I recommend adding lemon to most of the water you drink.

Hydration can also be assisted by eating more raw fruit and vegetables. Cooked food is often drier, pulling hydration from your body to assist digestion. Raw soups can be a good source of hydration as they often contain the right minerals to increase fluid absorption into the cells. Eating watermelon is also an excellent way to rehydrate.

Cucumber juice and coconut water are also very hydrating. You've seen that coconut water is also an antiviral, so it is a very good option. I generally drink a lot of vegetable juices; I find them not only hydrating but cleansing and energy-boosting, too. The *Medical Medium* books recommend drinking celery juice every day. I make various vegetable juice mixes and have them on hand in my fridge to drink daily.

The temperature of what you drink is also important. At Ayurvedic retreats, all liquids are served warm (even in 30-degree Indian heat). The kinds of liquids you drink include water with garlic, water with ginger, water with coriander seed, and water with various types of bark. Water is never consumed cold or plain – it always has something in it. These are not herbal teas as such – they are more like infused waters. Cold water is believed to imbalance your doshas. It constricts your blood vessels, and your body may not be able to absorb all the nutrients and vitamins from food. Warm water speeds up the digestion process and is even good for your gut health. Cold water also solidifies the fats from the food you eat and makes it tough for your body to break them down. If you do not like drinking warm water, at least try room-temperature water to keep your digestion in its optimal state.

Herbal teas are generally not as hydrating as other beverages but have many benefits. Allow the herbs to infuse in hot water, or put fresh herbs into water at room temperature and allow them to infuse for a few hours. I use a brand of herbs called Natural Products in

South Africa. These are available in various health stores but can be ordered online from Pharma Germania directly. Some of the herbs I drink are listed below, with my reasons for drinking them. I generally drink them at room temperature.

- Astragalus: Strengthens the immune system
- Indian celery seed: Joint pain and acidity in the joints
- Lemon balm: Anxiety and sleeplessness
- Passion flower: Anxiety and sleeplessness
- Chamomile: Calming and soothing, good for infection in the system
- Peppermint: Cleansing and refreshing, settles the stomach
- Valerian: PTSD and trauma
- St John's wort: Depression and difficulties with nerves
- Ginseng: Strengthens the immune system, assists with fatigue
- Ginger: Strengthens the immune system
- Liquorice root: Kills viruses, assists with fatigue
- Olive leaf: Strengthens the immune system
- Echinacea: Strengthens the immune system
- Gotu kola: Antimicrobial, anti-diabetic, anti-inflammatory, antidepressant, memory-enhancing properties
- Turmeric: Lowers inflammation.

Many of these you can also obtain in capsule format from the health shop, but it is likely that the absorption is better in the herbal tea format.

Alcohol is unfortunately your enemy. It is well known for promoting systemic inflammation and aggravating multiple health conditions. It creates an acidic state in the body, leaches essential nutrients from your system (like vitamin B), affects your sleep, blocks the liver and detoxification pathways, weakens the immune system, and its sugar content causes an array of issues. Some people with autoimmunity I have met and worked with have a strong aversion to alcohol; others have a close friendship with it and use it to manage symptoms such as anxiety and pain. It provides some relief in the moment, but often this comes at a price of ever-increasing symptoms. Some of my clients tell me that they wake up feeling inflamed and depressed anyway, so what difference does it make if they drink or not? I can understand that way of thinking, but I encourage you to work with this and shift it. What you are doing with alcohol is coping, and coping means you are blocking difficult emotions – allow these to surface and let them be a guide to what you need to heal inside you or change around you.

While coffee is purported to have a number of health benefits, due to the severe acidity it creates in the body, and the knock-on effect of this on inflammation, cut it out. You may experience a withdrawal or detox period, so this may need to be done gradually and only once your detoxification pathways are working better. Caffeine in coffee and tea can prevent us from resting when we should, and this can put our bodies in a fight-or-flight setting instead of a rest-and-digest setting. Caffeine is known to interfere with sleep; because most of our liver detoxifying and healing takes place when we're sleeping, we want to avoid anything that may interfere with sleep. We want to give the body every opportunity to heal. Caffeine also weakens the adrenals and can increase gut permeability.

Black tea, green tea and any other stimulating drinks should be cut out too and replaced with herbal tea. If you are craving a similar replacement, I recommend drinking maca, cacao and medicinal mushroom lattes. I use a mushroom powder that includes a blend of reishi, shiitake, chaga, cordyceps and lion's mane, as well as maca powder, cacao powder, coconut oil and a bit of honey to taste in coconut milk.

Eliminate all carbonated soft drinks from your diet. These generally have high levels of sugar and certain acids, both of which can be harmful to your health. Overconsumption may harm oral health through dental erosion, as well as other major health issues such obesity, raised blood glucose levels and an increased risk of disease.

Drinking poor-quality water can be a health risk – the very substance you need most to detox could be the one adding the toxins. Water quality is measured by several factors, such as the concentration of dissolved oxygen, bacteria levels, the amount of salt (or salinity), or the amount of material suspended in the water (turbidity). In some bodies of water, the concentration of microscopic algae and quantities of pesticides, herbicides, heavy metals and other contaminants may also be measured to determine water quality. Where I live, the tap water has a very low quality, which leaves me with the option of drinking water out of plastic containers. If you have natural resources of water around, seek them out. If you are unsure about the quality of your tap water, filter and boil it before drinking.

The primary risk of drinking bottled water is exposure to harmful toxins from the plastic. BPA and other plastic toxins can then make their way into your bloodstream, which can cause a host of problems including various cancers as well as liver and kidney damage. When buying bottled water, always go for glass if you can. Look at the label and consider the pH of the water – this should be about 7,25–7,35 (the normal range in a healthy body). Mineral content should also be considered, with a preference for low fluoride and copper (especially if you have thyroid difficulties). It should be sourced from a natural place. Carbonated or sparkling water sometimes have salt added to improve their taste. Sometimes small amounts of other minerals are included. Natural sparkling mineral waters do exist, such as Perrier and San Pellegrino, but these are often expensive. Carbon dioxide and water react chemically to produce carbonic acid, a weak acid that's been shown to stimulate the same nerve receptors in your mouth as mustard. This triggers a burning, prickly sensation that can be both irritating and enjoyable. The pH of carbonated water is 3–4, which means it's slightly acidic and thus may not be ideal for healing and detoxification. One of the biggest concerns about sparkling water is its effect on your teeth, as your enamel is directly exposed to acid. Interestingly, a carbonated drink may enhance digestion by improving swallowing ability and reducing constipation.

Supplements

We can think of taking supplements as a way of getting the biochemistry in your body back in order. Ideally, you should be getting this diverse nutrition from food, but this may not always be possible with our lifestyles and the quality of food available.

If you are going to take supplements, only take good-quality ones as low-quality ones could expose you to toxins. Please check the ingredients of your supplements and research what they are if you are not sure. Supplements containing magnesium stearate, a binding agent, are not recommended as this ingredient does not support absorption. Always read the labels and evaluate what is inside. Price doesn't always equate to quality. Some of your vitamin and mineral balances can be tested via blood tests. Functional medical practitioners typically test iron, vitamin D, vitamin B12 and magnesium levels. This is a good place to start as you can begin to see what, if any, imbalances need to be corrected. Certain supplements should not be taken unless indicated by deficiencies that come up in blood tests.

Some people prefer to take vitamin drips. This proves very effective for those with gut issues, who may struggle to absorb nutrients from food or supplementation. Please check if you are deficient via blood tests before doing these drips, as delivering high-dose vitamins intravenously can be hard on the liver and could cause damage to various organs. Various drips are available and ones to consider include multivitamin (especially vitamin B), iron and glutathione. Nicotinamide adenine dinucleotide (NAD) IVs have been proposed for managing autoimmune conditions. For some people, these IVs may overstimulate the system.

You may need to vary your supplements by listening to your body's symptoms and needs. There is a danger of putting things out of balance with supplements – for example, too much vitamin D may give you heart palpitations, and too much iron may damage many of your organs. Be aware of the side effects and when readjustment may be required.

A good place to start is with some foundational, immune system supporting and detoxifying supplements including vitamin C, vitamin B complex (specifically vitamin B12), zinc, selenium, vitamin D3, iron, magnesium glycinate, L-lysine, NAD, glutathione, curcumin, a good probiotic and quercetin. A spore probiotic may be preferable to an ordinary one as it is more resistant to stomach pH, stable at room temperature and delivers a greater quantity of high-viability bacteria to the small intestine. It is best to take these supplements individually for now as multivitamins may contain constituents like soya that may not be beneficial for you.

- Vitamin C is an important part of the immune system, which defends against viruses, bacteria and other pathogens. Food sources of vitamin C include oranges, tomatoes (if these can work for you), strawberries, papaya, mango, cauliflower and lemon. Liposomal vitamin C may be more efficiently absorbed by the body. This is a form of vitamin C delivered in fat bubbles called liposomes, which protect the vitamin's pathway through the digestive system into the bloodstream.

- Vitamin B12 is an important B vitamin and is linked to almost all autoimmune diseases. A deficiency can lead to a number of symptoms and can even progress to neurological issues if left untreated. It occurs naturally in animal products like meat and eggs, so it is not available in a vegetarian diet.

- Zinc helps your immune system and metabolism to function. It is also important for wound healing and your sense of taste and smell. Foods rich in zinc include shellfish, especially oysters, crab and lobster, beef, poultry, pork, legumes, nuts, seeds and whole grains.

- Selenium is an antioxidant that helps lower oxidative stress in your body, which reduces inflammation and enhances immunity. Foods containing selenium include Brazil nuts, seafood and meats. Selenium is a very important supplement for thyroid problems.

- Vitamin D3 is an anti-inflammatory and antioxidant, and has neuroprotective properties that support immune health, muscle function and brain cell activity. Food sources include salmon, trout, eggs and cod liver oil.

- Iron is needed for your body to produce haemoglobin, which helps red blood cells carry oxygen throughout the body, and myoglobin, a protein that helps provide oxygen to the cells in your muscles. Iron is regarded as a heavy metal so there is contrary information about it enhancing the growth and virulence of pathogens. However, the body's immune system uses iron – it is necessary for the activation and proliferation of immune cells – and a higher oxygen content in the blood lowers viral load. Foods high in iron include shellfish, spinach, liver and other organ meats, legumes, red meat, pumpkin seeds, quinoa, broccoli and fish. Iron should only be supplemented when doing so is indicated by blood tests, as excess iron is dangerous in the body.

- Magnesium glycinate may help lower blood pressure and reduce stroke, cardiovascular disease and type 2 diabetes risks, improve bone health and prevent migraines. It helps maintain normal heart rhythms and relieves anxiety. In research, certain conditions have been shown to improve with magnesium supplementation, including fibromyalgia and chronic fatigue syndrome. The best food sources include dark-green leafy vegetables, nuts and seeds, beans and fruit such as bananas and blackberries. When possible, always opt for foods grown in healthy soils that are local and organic. These soils contain the highest concentration of nutrients and minerals. Magnesium L-threonate is another, often preferred, option for magnesium supplementation as it is believed to be easily absorbed by the body.

- L-lysine is a foundational amino acid. As a supplement it is a powerful weapon against viruses. It hinders and stops all herpes viruses. It impairs the ability of viral cells to move and reproduce. The *Medical Medium* describes it as the powder that comes out of a fire extinguisher – a viral retardant that deters viruses from proliferating. L-lysine strengthens the immune system in the liver and aids in some of the organ's most important functions. It acts as an anti-inflammatory to the entire nervous system, especially the CNS and the vagus and phrenic nerves. This is because it inhibits and reduces viral loads, which means fewer viral neurotoxins are produced to inflame the nervous system. Potatoes, kiwis, apples, cherries and pears contain L-lysine and are helpful to include regularly in your diet.

- NAD works to repair and boost your mitochondrial energy system found in every cell of the body. As we age, we see a gradual decline in cellular NAD levels. This is linked to numerous age-associated diseases. Some potential strategies that boost NAD levels include lifestyle changes, such as increasing exercise, reducing caloric intake, eating a healthy diet, and following a consistent daily circadian rhythm pattern through healthy sleeping habits and mealtimes.

- Glutathione is a powerful antioxidant that helps to

metabolise toxins, break down free radicals and support immune function. Food sources include broccoli, cauliflower, cabbage, onion, garlic, avocado, squash and spinach.

- Curcumin assists in wound healing and post-operative, neuropathic, arthritic and joint pain. It is a powerful anti-inflammatory, with anti-tumour, antiparasitic and antibiotic properties. It is found in turmeric.

- As you've seen, probiotics promote a healthy digestive tract and immune system.

- Quercetin boosts immunity, fights inflammation and alleviates allergies. Fruits and vegetables that have high amounts of quercetin include apples, kale, tomatoes, broccoli, raw asparagus, raw red onion, nuts, seeds and red grapes. Quercetin is also in herbs such as American elder, St John's wort and *Ginkgo biloba*.

Lesser-known additional supplements that you may want to add include the following:

- Fulvic acid, which reduces inflammation, delivers usable oxygen to cells providing electrolytes and trace minerals, boosts metabolism, supports the circulatory system, improves brain function, memory, mood and heart health, removes toxins and heavy metals, regenerates cells, helps with nutrient absorption, repopulates gut flora, and helps to balance hormones. It is found in vegetables.

- Serrapeptase, an enzyme that breaks down biofilms. When bacteria and viruses chronically overwhelm the body, biofilms are involved – mucous membranes that wrap around a clump of bacteria, viruses and fungi and inhibit the immune system from attacking and clearing them out. Serrapeptase breaks this biofilm down and exposes these pathogens for elimination by your immune system.

- Activated charcoal, a processed form of common charcoal that contains pores that can trap other chemicals and prevent them from being absorbed by the body. It is used to treat certain types of chemical poisoning and has also been used in alternative medicine to treat gas and indigestion. It is very useful during autoimmune flare-ups, especially when the flare-up is linked to eating something that the system doesn't agree with.

- Coenzyme Q10 (CoQ10), an antioxidant that your body produces naturally. Your cells use it for growth and maintenance. It is found in meat, fish and nuts.

- Resveratrol, a chemical mostly found in red grapes and grape products (wine and juice). It may have many effects in the body, including expanding blood vessels and reducing blood clotting.

- N-acetylcysteine (NAC), which produces antioxidants and replenishes glutathione.

- Diatomaceous earth, a unique type of sand that consists of fossilised algae. Please ensure that you only ingest the food-grade version of this. It is a concentrated form of silica, and it may assist with cleansing and restoring the digestive tract, improving bone, hair and nail growth, and flushing parasites out. It is believed to open up the biofilms of parasites.

ৡৄ

Herbs

There are herbs out there to treat almost every symptom. Herbs may help your detoxification pathways, help you fight or rid yourself of pathogens, support various organs or systems in your body, strengthen your immune system, calm the mind, alleviate specific symptoms, and provide nutritional support to create homeostatic balance in the body.

Whenever you need to consider taking a medication, remember that there is often a herbal alternative. Herbs are slower-acting and need to be used over the long term to be effective. Some herbs interact with each other or medication in an uncomfortable or even dangerous way – for example, St John's wort cannot be combined with antidepressant medication, as this overstimulates serotonin increase in the brain and can have dangerous consequences. If in doubt, stick to the basics, follow your intuition and, most importantly, check in with an integrative doctor or other holistic practitioner.

Immune-boosting and virus- and parasite-fighting herbs

- Astragalus is an immune booster that helps diabetes, as a heart tonic and in anaemia. It increases the white blood cell count and has anti-cancer properties. It acts as a tonic to protect the immune system, aids adrenal gland function and digestion, increases metabolism, produces spontaneous sweating, promotes healing, and provides energy to combat fatigue and prolonged stress and increase stamina.

- Echinacea is a helpful immune booster as it stimulates certain white blood cells. It has antibiotic and antiviral qualities.

- Ginseng is an adaptogen that assists with energy/fatigue, depression, diabetes, withstanding stress, mental alertness, colds and flu, improves overall health, reduces cholesterol, and lowers blood pressure. It is also an aphrodisiac. It strengthens the adrenal and reproductive glands, enhances immune function, promotes lung functioning and stimulates the appetite. Ginseng also assists with enhancing mitochondrial function. Ginseng interacts with many medications, so please consult with your doctor before taking it.

- Olive leaf has antioxidant, antibacterial, antimicrobial, anti-inflammatory and immune stimulating properties. It can be used for chronic fatigue, arthritis, psoriasis, anxiety and fever. It has strong antiviral properties and is used in holistic medicine to treat certain viruses.

- Cat's claw is believed to fight various viruses. It also balances an overactive immune system. It can help a variety of health conditions, including viral infections (such as herpes, HPV and HIV), Alzheimer's disease, cancer, arthritis, diverticulitis, peptic ulcers, colitis, gastritis, haemorrhoids, parasites and leaky gut syndrome.

- Liquorice root is considered one of the world's oldest herbal remedies. It has potent antioxidant, anti-inflammatory and antimicrobial effects. It may ease upper respiratory infections, treat ulcers and aid digestion. It fights inflammation and viral, bacterial and parasitic infections. It also energises the system, helping chronic fatigue and burnout.

- Taheebo or pau d'arco reduces inflammation, assists in fighting pathogens and helps with mitochondrial function.

- Wormwood has been used for medicinal purposes for thousands of years, and in making absinthe. It is used to treat worms and parasites – it appears to cause parasites to lose muscle function and die. It also increases stomach acidity and helps produce saliva, so it helps digestion. It is useful for migraines. A compound found in wormwood called artemisinin may limit the body's inflammatory cytokine production. *Artemisia annua* (sweet wormwood) has been widely used to treat autoimmune diseases such as SLE and RA in TCM. A perfect formula for parasite cleansing includes a combination of black walnut, quassia, cloves and wormwood, alongside the use of diatomaceous earth.

- Four medicinal mushrooms for treating viruses stand out. Penicillin was the first true antibiotic that was discovered back in 1928 and is a fungus, just like a mushroom. Mushrooms have their medicinal origins in TCM. They are:

  - Reishi, known as the mushroom of immortality in TCM. Research has shown its activity against various viruses.

  - Cordyceps, a legendary natural medicine found in parts of Asia (originally Tibet), increases ATP levels and oxygen utilisation by the body, resulting in an increase of useful energy.

  - Maitake, which helps to fight off the influenza virus and boosts the body's supply of antiviral cytokines. It is classified as an adaptogen, a substance that balances the immune system and helps the body to resist the negative effects of stress.

- Shiitake, which may stop the replication of viruses.

Detoxification herbs

Herbs and supplements that support the detoxification process include spirulina, chlorella, NAC, glutathione, aloe, activated charcoal, milk thistle and Warburgia. Spirulina and chlorella are specifically for detoxing (or chelating) heavy metals out of the body. Spirulina, moringa, barley grass, pitaya powder, cat's claw and ashwagandha can be put into smoothies as they often come in powder form. NAC and glutathione enhance the functioning of the detoxification pathways in the body. Aloe (ferox) cleans the gut. Activated charcoal absorbs toxins from the gut to be expelled. Milk thistle cleans the liver. Warburgia cleans the kidneys.

Nervous system regulating herbs

Herbs and supplements to calm the adrenals down may be useful in a dysregulated individual. This may give the immune system the space to come back online. The following herbs may assist in calming the system, but they also have additional benefits:

- Lemon balm: A carminative, nervine, antispasmodic, antidepressant, diaphoretic, antimicrobial and hepatic. It is appropriate for neuralgia, anxiety-induced palpitations, insomnia and migraines associated with tension. It has a tonic effect on the heart and circulatory system, and lowers blood pressure. It has some hormone-regulating effects.
- St John's wort: Has a sedative and pain-relieving effect. It

can be used for treatment of neuralgia, anxiety, tension and similar problems. It is especially appropriate for use when menopausal changes trigger irritability and anxiety. It also treats mild to moderate depression, insomnia, neuralgia and hysteria, and helps fight viral infections. This cannot be taken when using antidepressant medications.

- Valerian: Acts as a sedative, improves circulation and reduces mucus from colds. Treats anxiety, insomnia, high blood pressure, depression, stress and tension.

- Chamomile: Has anti-inflammatory, antispasmodic, antibacterial and antifungal properties. Helps with nausea, insomnia, muscular pain, colic and nervous disorders, and is useful as a mouthwash.

- Ashwagandha: As you've seen, ashwagandha is widely used in Ayurvedic medicine. It is an ingredient of many formulations prescribed for musculoskeletal conditions such as arthritis and rheumatism, and is used as a general adaptogen to increase energy, improve overall health and balance pathological states. It is credited with enhancing the body's resilience to stress, preventing adrenal exhaustion, balancing hormones and enhancing the function of the brain and nervous system.

Here is a short list of some of the common symptoms that come up in autoimmune conditions, and some supplement and herb combinations that may help with these:

- Nerve pain: Vitamin B12, St Johns' wort, lemon balm, curcumin
- Back pain: Vitamin B12, valerian, magnesium, curcumin
- Seizures: Vitamin B6, magnesium, vitamin E, manganese,

omega-3, chamomile, valerian, passion flower, kava, *Bacopa monnieri*

- Anxiety and panic attacks: Valerian, lemon balm, passion flower, ashwagandha, magnesium, gamma-aminobutyric acid (GABA)
- Constipation: Aloe
- Depression: St John's wort (does not combine with antidepressant medication), saffron, Vitamin B12, eating and smelling citrus, turmeric, anti-inflammatory diet
- Headaches: Vitamin B2, magnesium, vitamin D, coenzyme Q10, chamomile, lavender, peppermint oil (topically)
- Sleep problems: Melatonin, valerian, lemon balm, passion flower, chamomile
- Migraines: Vitamin B2, magnesium, coenzyme Q10, feverfew, valerian, coriander seed, butterbur, willow, ginger, peppermint oil (topically)
- Cysts: Omega-3, chasteberry, shatavari
- Hormonal imbalances: Black cohosh, dong quai, ashwagandha, red clover, milk thistle, shatavari, doing a liver cleanse
- Endometriosis: Shatavari, vitamin B6, magnesium, omega-3, curcumin, ginger, cramp bark, calendula, chasteberry, chamomile, pine bark, peppermint
- Joint pain and costochondritis: Indian celery seed, L-lysine, curcumin, ginger, eucalyptus, Boswellia, collagen powder, cat's claw
- Hair loss: Iron, vitamin B12, silica, collagen, diatomaceous earth
- Tinnitus: L-lysine, *Gingko biloba*, zinc, vitamin B12,

melatonin, flavonoids
- Eye floaters: Vitamin C, curcumin, MSM, vitamin D, L-lysine, milk thistle, *Gingko biloba*
- Teeth-chattering, jaw weakness or tightness, body vibration: Valerian, chamomile
- Nausea: Ginger, activated charcoal
- Burnout (which is often linked to chronic fatigue caused by an increased viral load): Ginseng, liquorice root, ashwagandha
- Kidney infections: Warburgia, cranberry extract, marshmallow root, parsley.

Regulating yourself

If most people with an autoimmune condition were in the wild and a lion attacked them, they would do what they do best: go into a freeze response. This response is the most familiar of the fight, flight, freeze triad for you, as it is likely where you spent a fair amount of time in your childhood. Here are a few tips for starting to ease yourself out of the freeze response: allow connection and daily human-to-human interaction; co-regulate with nature and animals; lower your level of daily stimulation and intensity; commit to short moments in which you can pause and anchor yourself in the present; nurture your passions, preferences and needs; and be patient and kind about where you are – practice self-compassion.

Autoimmune flare-ups are primarily the result of psychological and physical stress on the body, or diet and allergens. When I was at the start of my healing journey, the smallest emotional event, like an argument or even watching a thriller, would flare my body up. Studies have found that up to 80 per cent of patients reported significant and 'uncommon emotional stress' before their initial disease onset. Your flare-ups may be triggered by current events that resemble your trauma history. If there is a pattern in your life originating from your relationship with your mother of being taken advantage of, for example, it could be that when this happens in the present your body launches into a cascade of symptoms. Your body is responding to the emotions behind the whole trauma chain, and not just the present event. Often, there is even attachment trauma behind this, from our very early years. There is often a chronic feeling of being unsafe that pops up with this triggering. So, the most important thing we can do in these situations is create safety, grounding and connection. It is good to have a ritual for creating safety. First, slow down. Try to reduce the number of things you have to do to a minimum. You want to reduce the arousal in your body to an absolute minimum.

Another way to create safety is to talk ourselves down from our triggers. We may need to reassure ourselves that we are safe, that we are not alone. This may need external evidence, and the best way to do this is to engage with our social network (or, in somatic psychology language, to activate the social engagement system). This may mean finding the family members, friends, therapists, healers or animals that make us feel safe and connected. The people to whom we feel attuned and who show us empathy will switch our system into safe mode.

In *The Power of Now*, Eckhart Tolle writes that our problems are rooted in our identification with our minds – and that we should become aware of the present moment instead of losing ourselves in fear and worry about the past or present. Bringing our awareness to the present can bring us out of that overwhelmed place – perhaps saying to yourself, 'Right now, I am okay.' Our monkey minds can take over with restless, unsettled and confused thoughts. Often, these thoughts are tied to our inner critic.

Another thing a friend once told me to do is 'be where your feet are'. Often, just looking down at your feet can bring you back into the present moment. Use meditation and mindfulness, in which you become intensely aware of what you are sensing and feeling in the moment, without interpretation or judgement. Practising mindfulness may include breathing methods (more about this later) and guided imagery (see the safe space exercise a little later).

Crossing the cerebral hemispheres is very useful, as demonstrated in psychotherapies such as eye movement desensitisation and reprocessing (EMDR – see Bessel van der Kolk's *The Body Keeps the Score* for more about this), and Ayurvedic therapies such as shirodhara. This switches off the amygdala. A technique that may be useful is alternating between humming and counting. Some people find it effective just to look from side to side and notice something on each side. Another way of doing this is to wear earphones that send a tone or soothing sound into alternating ears. Moving a wand, finger or even a pen back and forth from left to right may also do the trick. Touch or vibration on alternating hands is another strategy, if you have someone nearby to help you.

The vagus nerve can also be stimulated or toned through breathing exercises (long, slow inhalations through the nose, and even longer, slower exhalations through the mouth; alternate nostril breathing), humming, chanting, gargling, singing, massage and exercise.

The most ideal solution, which may not be available to us too often, is to go into nature to or a retreat centre and find our ground again. These are places that are quiet and gentle, which can slowly shift us out of our adrenal state – places that force you to be still and reflect.

I have found a few techniques effective for managing the fight-or-flight response in the moment:

- Trauma Release Exercises (TRE): A sequence of yoga-like exercises that helps release the psoas muscle and deeply held tension, stress and fear. It helps you access your body's ability to tremor or shake trauma out.
- Legs up the wall: A yoga pose that is known to be restorative and help aid relaxation.
- Grounding: Place your feet in the grass or on the soil and connect with the earth. Engage the senses – notice what you see, hear, taste, feel and smell around you.
- Venting negative emotions: Scream as loudly as you can and, if possible, cry (if screaming is not possible, imagine yourself screaming); punch a pillow or hit it with a stick, or invest in a punching bag; pound your fists on a table; write it all down in a journal; collapse and sob for an hour; try yoga.
- Emotional freedom technique (EFT) or tapping: Tapping on meridian points on the body while saying affirmations helps release emotions stored in the body. There are many videos on YouTube that demonstrate this.

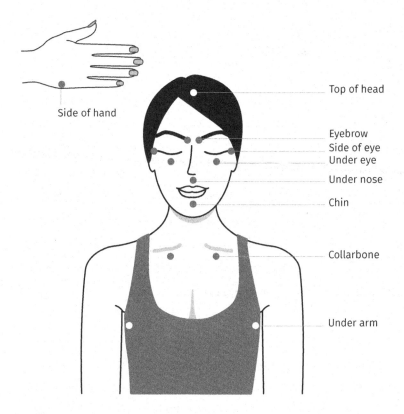

Side of hand

Top of head

Eyebrow
Side of eye
Under eye

Under nose

Chin

Collarbone

Under arm

Whenever you get lost in all your stress, remember to identify your resources. A resource is an internal focal point to which you can return when that too-much feeling comes over you. It can range from a soothing, calming image, feeling or sensation to an actual person who evokes the same feelings of safety and security, as long as it is something positive in your life. These can be positive character traits of yours, beautiful memories, experiences you have had, people or animals you have enjoyed in your life, your accomplishments, a possession you value, an amazing movie character who resonates with you, or anything that comes up and floods you with a positive energy. Write these down and have them on hand: when we get into our more difficult mindsets, it is often challenging to conjure up our resources.

The shamanic way, the way of humans when we still lived in tribes, was to sing, dance and drum. Often, just putting music on can shift you into a different mindset (and no, heavy metal is not likely going to do the trick here!). Country music and Disney music has been shown to move people into an optimal arousal space, as they seem to activate the parasympathetic nervous system. People often report a sense of invigoration and euphoria when using their voice to sing. When we allow ourselves the joy of self-expression through our voices, it awakens parts of us that may have been dormant or neglected our entire lives. Dancing – the way your body needs to, an expressive dancing, rather – may be just what you need to dislodge frozen emotion and trauma. People often report a sense of flow and aliveness after they have had a good dancing session.

Often, thinking about home can be very soothing and grounding. If there isn't a home that feels right for you to think about, bring into your mind what home would be like if it was ideal for you. Home is where our roots are, and roots mean safety. If it needs to be a fantasy home, so be it. And you can follow up with the exercise below; maybe the two will tie in …

 Task

My safe space

Bring to mind a place that feels safe for you. It can be anywhere in the world, any place you choose. A beach, a mountain, at home, anywhere. This is your sanctuary, a place you can escape to any time you want to. Start visualising your sanctuary and all the detail in it. This is a place where you can completely relax. Imagine what this place needs for you to feel calm and at ease.

Start with the physical layout. Look around you ... let's notice any sights in this place. Notice the colours, shapes, objects, the changes in light, notice textures, notice movement. Are there buildings, or trees? Are you indoors or outdoors? Is it large or small? Is it night or day? How are you responding to the things you see? Are certain things you see bringing up memories? Who is in this place? Are you alone? Let's imagine all the beautiful detail that makes your place enjoyable. Take this in for a few moments.

Now, turn your attention to the things you hear around you. Can you hear birds, maybe some waves crashing or people talking? Can you hear animals? Is there music? Even silence has a sound ... a resonance. Are there sounds you are responding to in a particular way? Are the sounds soothing and comforting you? Listen to the sounds for a moment ...

Now, imagine any smells that your place has to offer – are the smells intense? Can you smell coffee, incense, perfume, the ocean, flowers, or a fire burning? Does it smell fresh? What are the smells making you think about? Take a few moments to focus on the smells ...

Imagine any sensations of touch. Are you touching anything in your sanctuary? Anything you are sitting on? What is the temperature? Is there a breeze?

Now, imagine any tastes. Are you perhaps tasting anything? Are you eating or drinking? What does it taste like? What does it remind you of? Experience this for a moment ...

What else are you doing in your sanctuary? Maybe you are resting, reading a book, sleeping? Maybe you are taking a walk ...

Now, see your sanctuary in totality, as you have designed it. This is your safe space. A place you can come to whenever the world becomes too distressing. A place that can give you a temporary break from reality in your imagination. Picture yourself here for a few moments ... Imagine a feeling of calm and peace. You have no worries or concerns in this place, where you can rejuvenate, relax and enjoy just being.

Memorise the sights, sounds, sensations around you. Know that you can return to this place in your mind whenever you need a break. You can take a mental vacation and allow yourself to relax and regroup before returning to your regular role in life. Take a snapshot of this place that you can use to remind yourself about this relaxed feeling.

If you have some time, draw this sanctuary for yourself and put the picture up somewhere where stress visits you often.

A further exercise could be to create a safety ritual for yourself: often, when we are in a tunnel of stress, we may find it difficult to direct ourselves to what can regulate us.

Energy audit

Preventing burnout is important for maintaining regulation. An energy audit is a balance sheet of what you are doing to bring energy into your life, and what is pulling energy out of your life. Consider all the inflows of energy into your life, as well as all the outflows. Perhaps a good activity would be to make a table of these inflows and outflows. This may involve looking at all the people around you and the interactions you have with them, all the activities you do, and how you spend your time in general.

When we are in a state of depletion, we either find ways to give to ourselves, or we sometimes end up taking from others. Determine the things that make you feel better or worse energy-wise. Maintaining this energy audit so that there are more inflows that outflows will require you to have healthy boundaries with yourself and others. Healthy boundaries mean making self-care a priority, setting limits for yourself, and learning to say no to opportunities and requests that may overextend you.

While you are healing, plan for doing more of what makes you feel better. For autoimmune conditions, things that make you feel better may be sleeping, spending time with loved ones, being in nature, walking, massage, reading, sitting on a beach, being warm, hugging and yoga. Things that could make you feel worse include lack of sleep, being stressed, overworking, being around negative people, fighting with loved ones, lack of sunshine, cold weather, being in traffic, intense exercise, caffeine and drinking alcohol.

Connection

We humans are wired to be social beings and connection is a daily need to be fulfilled. From an evolutionary standpoint, part of our survival depended on our ability to be connected socially within our communities. Social rejection and alienation may contribute to alterations of stress, thyroid and other hormone levels. In an experiment, baby rats were denied both connection and nutrition. When they were given access to both these elements again, they went towards the connection first – they moved towards sources of social energy before they fed themselves, even when they were bordering on starvation. 'All you need is love' – those famous words from the Beatles song couldn't be truer.

When something compromises our sense of survival in the world (finances, perhaps), our sense of purpose (a feeling of serving this world in some way), or our sense of belonging, we go into a fight-or-flight state, trying to restore or preserve that thing we sense we are losing. Next, we go into a depression or shut down when we feel we may be losing the fight. Belonging in an evolutionary sense means survival. I personally don't believe in introversion – I think of it as a reaction to trauma when people need to isolate as they are triggered in social company by their trauma history, which becomes draining, making them want to stay away. If you are struggling in the space of connection, it may be worth investigating whether traumatic experiences in your history are creating barriers to connection. What has happened with friends, in romance and with family, which could be making you keep your distance from people?

When we are raised in inconsistent environments in childhood, we may seek out similar inconsistency later in life, unconsciously repeating patterns. Environments with intermittent reinforcement are addictive and have a greater hold than consistent environments.

Important to discuss here is the negative connections we may form in life. There are energetic links between you and everyone with whom you engage. Your vibration affects and is affected by the vibration around you. If you find yourself having recurring thoughts about someone, it may be that energetic link in action. Sometimes we are exposed to toxic relationships or encounters, and that energy may drain us, especially if we begin to play the role of the pleaser, the fixer, or the responsible one. It may also be that those recurring thoughts are part of the action of PTSD. Your brain keeps repeating a trauma memory, which makes the person occupy a lot of space in your mind. The symptoms of unhealthy attachments may come up as depleted energy levels, obsessive thoughts about another person, regularly speaking about that person, unexplained depression, lowered immune function, and unusual addictive behaviours and character aspects. This energy drain may mean that your system no longer has the vitality to fight the pathogens you are being exposed to. If you are sensitive to this, you may need to cleanse or protect yourself regularly. Wearing black stones such as tourmaline or onyx on the skin may help with protection. Bathing in the sea, Epsom salts or Himalayan salt, or using incense (especially sage), can be a form of cleansing, but you can design your own rituals that make you feel clear. Consider your boundaries to protect your space from these energies. Kelly Brogan states that when we are ready to walk away from a person who does not meet our needs, we own the fact that we have needs and we stop meeting them externally by being cooperative and giving into this secure illusion of safety. This breeds a power inside us that can move us towards true individuation.

Find connections that are consistent, healthy and reliable. Healthy connection makes us feel safe and helps us relax, and we heal relationally. One good relationship can re-regulate your ANS and erase the negative beliefs that may have originated in a traumatic one – it can help reset trauma. Just being around some of my friends has filled me with nurturing that has done wonders for my nervous system. Let the autoimmunity guide you towards those who feel good for you in your body.

Invited physical touch such as hugs, comfort, warmth and nurturing all make the adrenals less active. My autoimmune patients often report feeling a lot better at the start of a new relationship. The release of oxytocin may pacify the adrenal response that is driving their condition. You've seen that in autoimmune conditions there has been deprivation of social and emotional needs, and that sufferers are drawn energetically to people who replay this. Often it is better to be alone than in the company of family members who deny the illness, perhaps, or exacerbate it with their own demands, pulling you into dynamics where you need to be the fixer, carer, pleaser or supporter. It is important to step out of this dynamic if it is the case for you. Sometimes we cannot step out of this so easily, and we need to use communication and boundaries to manage the dynamics that we repeatedly get pulled into. Be open, honest and vulnerable in your communications as others are not mind-readers and may not understand what you are experiencing and what you need. Stand firm in your boundaries and needs. Own your ultimatums. Don't take the bait of maintaining an unhealthy connection over keeping your own authenticity. When we stand firm in our needs, our trust of self grows. As you engage with your journey of healing and change, the kinds of people you attract into your life will change. According to Buddhism, one should choose 'noble' people as friends. What does this 'noble' mean for you?

Finding support in community or with a healer of some sort may be important. Having an invisible autoimmune condition can make you feel completely and utterly alone. Autoimmunity is very isolating. The lifestyle changes may be alienating, as suddenly you cannot eat certain things or consume alcohol. While friends and family members often rally around those with visible injuries or potentially terminal diagnoses like cancer, most are not gifted with the understanding of how to support someone who, according to them, looks largely healthy. Illness may also create a strain on certain relationships in that it forces a rebalance of roles and responsibilities. My clients often mention feelings of guilt for being a burden on their families, especially financially. Clear communication is key. People may not understand your symptoms or why you are seeking treatments that go against the grain of conventional medicine. But many others have gone through the same challenges and can help support you through yours. Whether a trusted friend, an online forum, a coach or a therapist, find someone who will listen to you and be supportive. Recognise that illness also has the potential to drive connection and compassion.

I know how scary this is. But you are not alone, and it's going to be okay. Feeling part of a community is a key aspect of the healing experience. There are Facebook groups out there for people with similar conditions – join them and connect. Training programmes such as Chronic Fatigue School offer both knowledge and a support base in a course format. Listening to podcasts about autoimmunity, the immune system and trauma may also create a sense of solidarity in all of this and have the added benefit of all the valuable information. (But please be careful with trauma podcasts, as they can be quite triggering and dysregulating.) Increased supportive social relationships, exposure to a context that favours healing behaviours and cultivation of a sense of meaning through engaging with others about your health will set you on a good path on this journey.

We exist in invisible bonds of an infinite network of connections: simple and complicated, direct or hidden, strong or delicate, temporary or very long-lasting. A web of connections, infinite but locally fragile, with and among everything – all beings. Most transformation and healing processes move you from disconnection to a sense of connection with yourself, others and the broader world (nature and cosmos). Everything about us – our brains or minds, and our bodies – is geared towards collaboration in social systems. This is our most powerful survival strategy, the key to our success as a species, and it is precisely this that breaks down in most forms of mental suffering. Relational traumas often involve the experience of being shamed or made to feel alone, defective, unwanted, worthless and unlovable.

Even relationships with other-than-human beings can bring a sense of love, care, trust, safety, universal connection and meaning into your life – God, animals, nature, spirits, guides, entities, angels, plant spirits, or whatever may resonate with you.

Connect – with everyone and everything.

Nature

Ancient cultures all had a strong link to their natural environments. In modern life, we seem to have lost this. Perhaps we need to consider our connection to plants, animals, the elements and even spirits. Spending time in nature, listening to the sound of ocean waves crashing or a river running can often bring us back into natural alignment. Fresh air, open spaces, natural beauty, calming sounds and immersion in the pulsating energies of nature are connected to increased feelings of well-being, including life satisfaction, vitality and happiness. By just allowing ourselves to become perceptive of the natural world around us, by hearing birds and the wind, we can draw ourselves into the present moment and connect with our own internal rhythms.

Think of yourself as a plant that needs the right conditions to thrive. Big-city lights, traffic and polluted air are certainly not the right conditions. As we step away from our devices and embrace nature – whether under a canopy of trees, on a wilderness trail, by a lake, on a beach, or in a green park – breathe in better air and soak up invisible energies, we become calmer, rejuvenated and restored, and these are excellent autoimmune healing strategies.

Natural soundscapes, such as the symphony of birds and trickling water, can positively influence human health, recent research has confirmed. Natural sounds improve health, increase positive affect and lower stress and annoyance. Data was collected from more than 7 500 people as part of the BBC series 'Forest 404', a podcast that depicts a world without nature. Participants reported that sounds of birdsong provided relief from stress and mental fatigue.

Many people with autoimmune conditions benefit from being near the sea. The sea heightens circulation and the immune system. Even inhaling sea mist is beneficial, as it contains negative ions. Negative ions help our bodies to absorb more oxygen, and they help regulate serotonin levels. Our pores may open, allowing our bodies to absorb trace elements and usher out toxins. The sea is also rich in iodine, a source that is gently stimulating and can assist the functioning of the thyroid. The ocean and swimming also stimulate the parasympathetic nervous system, resulting in a calm state, efficient organ function and a healthy brain–gut connection. Traveling to a tropical, sunny location invites low stress and an active lifestyle. These factors add to the benefits that are already being provided from the sun and ocean. They contribute to proper detoxification and overall wellness.

Getting some morning sun is a way of reconnecting with the natural world. Sunshine may improve vitamin D levels and assist in regulating circadian rhythms. Health-conscious Japanese people practice forest bathing. This entails spending time or strolling under a canopy of trees. Research shows that this can stimulate the production of natural killer (NK) cells, which improves immune strength and helps combat cancer. Rubber soles disconnect us from nourishing negative electrons and walking barefoot is a healing strategy. The earth's surface contains a limitless and continuously renewed supply of free electrons. Mounting evidence suggests that soaking up these negative electrons promotes optimal functioning of all body systems. Earthing, or grounding as it's sometimes called, reduces inflammation, lowers blood pressure, diminishes pain and improves immune response, fasting glucose and even sleep. Research shows that regular earthing may improve cardiovascular arrhythmias and autoimmune conditions like SLE, MS and RA.

When we get into nature, away from synthetic lights, we connect with our primitive rhythms and our circadian cycles synchronise. This helps our bodies function better. Increased vitamin D from sunlight supports better immune function, increased melatonin production from natural darkness leads to better sleep, and our stress hormone, cortisol, follows its natural pattern of rising in the morning and falling at night. Spending just a little time in nature has profound health benefits including improved immune function, increased NK cell function, reduced inflammation, lowered blood pressure, reduced pain, improved cardiovascular and respiratory systems, improved vitality and mood, reduced anxiety, better attention capacity, increased energy and faster recovery from illness and surgery.

Animals

I have seen many of my patients improve when they make contact with animals in some way. Animals can provide an experience of unconditional love in a time when other humans may not know what to do and say. Expose yourself to animals or get a pet if it feels right for you. Loving and caring for an animal floods your system with oxytocin. Consider whether the animal is going to be a stress or burden on you in terms of responsibility or finances.

An animal is often a good distractor and stress buffer, and can alleviate loneliness and provide comfort in difficult times. All animals are emotional support animals. I have witnessed many times, during online psychotherapy sessions, how animals gravitate to their owners when there is distress. There is certainly a form of unconditional support there. There are numerous studies confirming the positive mental health benefits of companion animals and, as we have seen, your mental health is your physical health too.

A dog may also promote physical activity and provide a sense of increased security. It is best not to get a busy or demanding breed of animal, as this may prove more stressful than valuable. I would carefully evaluate an animal if you are sourcing one from a shelter – as much as providing a safe and loving home to these animals may be very healing for them, the process of helping them recover from the trauma they may have experienced in their life before you may not be suitable for someone who needs to dedicate their resources to themselves. Worth considering also is that your immune system is not what it used to be, so it may be helpful to 'test' whether you are able to tolerate an animal's dander or whether you have some newfound sensitivities.

Rest and sleep

Sleep is affected by stress and trauma. If we don't sleep, our bodies' regenerative and healing capacity suffers. Most people see the recommended daily sleep of seven to eight hours as the target. But I think there is a greater truth about sleep. If you need more, you need to have more. My whole life I have preferred ten hours of sleep a night. When I was healing, my body would sometimes need extra naps – and sometimes, extra naps and too much sleep would make me feel worse. Intuition and listening to your body are the key. Generally, women need a bit more sleep than men.

Another important aspect of sleep is routine. Our bodies are happiest when we have a sleep routine. According to the most ancient traditions, we should rise and fall with the sun. In modern life this is near impossible, with so much activity being centred on the evenings. When you go to sleep at 9 p.m. or 10 p.m., you have better-quality sleep than if you go to sleep at midnight, so you often need a bit less sleep. Experiment with what your body feels it needs.

During the sleep cycle, your body initially goes into slow-wave sleep. It is believed that body regeneration takes place here. As the sleep cycle progresses, slow-wave sleep time shortens and REM sleep time starts lengthening. In REM sleep, memory consolidation takes place. It is the time of dreams, and when you are traumatised it is also when your mind may be healing. There are some theories that the integration and processing of the traumatic event takes place during this period.

Also worth considering when it comes to sleep is the Chinese body clock. According to this, every organ rejuvenates at a different time of the day or night. Some organs need a wake state to rejuvenate, and others need a sleep state. Many people in my practice tell me they wake up between 1 a.m. and 3 a.m. This is the time of the liver, which could indicate that their detoxification pathways have been affected in some way.

When I have been living in a state of autonomic dysregulation for some time, I know I need extra sleep until I balance myself. Going on holiday to hot environments often forces us to have the afternoon naps that we may need in addition to our normal sleep hours to replenish ourselves. A body and mind that is healing needs a lot of sleep – give this permission.

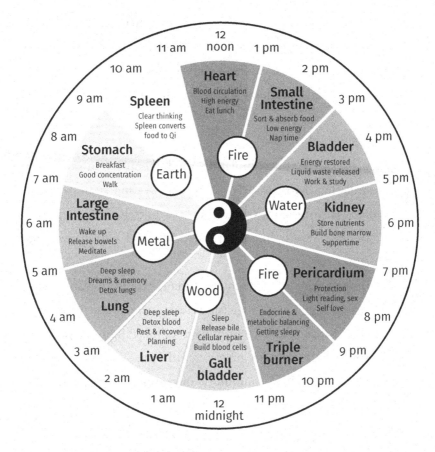

Often, I ask people who have sleep difficulties what they do before they sleep, and they tell me that they engage in an activity that could release quite a bit of adrenaline – being on their phone, watching television, working late – then rush off to bed and expect their system just to switch off. Consider easing the body into the sleep cycle. This may entail slowing down your whole way of being in the hours before bed.

Another word I need to mention here is stillness. This is a quality that most of us have forgotten, in this life of constant motion. Even while watching television, we could reach for our phones a dozen times. Be still – spend time just being. If this is hard because your mind is running wild, pulling you into a need to move or do something productive, confront this aspect of yourself. You are likely using your busy-ness as a way of avoiding internal discomfort and pain.

Exercise

Exercise is valuable for stimulating good chemistry in our brain and stimulating detoxification pathways. Sweating is an excellent way to lower your body's toxic burden. Exercise also improves mitochondrial health. Just don't overdo it, and please use good judgement.

A combination of stretching, strengthening, balance and aerobic exercise is most beneficial. Research shows that moderate-intensity physical exercises stimulate cellular immunity, while prolonged or high-intensity practices without appropriate rest can trigger decreased cellular immunity, increasing the propensity for infectious diseases. As a rule, you should feel more energised after these activities, not more tired.

When it comes to autoimmune conditions, the body may often not be in a state that can tolerate exercise very well. If you have chronic fatigue and run 10 kilometres you may feel better afterwards, but ultimately you are depleting yourself further. Running is something I often tell people to pause as it creates a similar adrenal response in the brain to being chased by a wild animal. This is not restorative. If your body needs healing, you may need to slow down instead of further aggravating your adrenals. The initial endorphin rush and detox of vigorous exercise may feel great, but the adrenals soon crash us and we feel worse than before, with higher adrenaline shutting down our immune system more and inviting further pathogens into our bodies. With autoimmune conditions you may find yourself more exhausted or more depleted than others even after a gentle yoga class. However, exercise is important, and the key is to find that sweet spot that stimulates flow in your body and doesn't leave you feeling worse.

I recommend doing more exercise that strengthens your core – the stronger your core, the more empowered and balanced you will feel, which will change your energy system. Considering weight training or strengthening exercise is important before our older years, as after age 50 you lose 1–2 per cent of muscle strength per year. Gentle daily walks may give your body the oxygenation it needs to fight pathogens and regenerate.

I also recommend taking up qigong, tai chi or yoga. These modalities are more than just exercise, and are a way of learning to move energy around your body and thus heal yourself. Qigong and tai chi are ancient self-healing systems. Qigong teaches you to feel and be aware of the energy flow in your body. Tai chi is similar but involves more movement. There is a reason why you see many older people gravitating towards this – it has a strong impact on restoring life force.

There are various yoga poses that stimulate the vagus nerve – many of the ones that require you to open your heart space have that effect. The breathing practice of yoga – pranayama – can be especially useful as some of these breathing techniques may help with regulating the autonomic nervous system. Om mantra chanting causes various changes in brain, having neurophysiological, neurochemical and neuroelectrical effects. Research shows that brain wave activity is affected by chanting Om. Chanting mantras silently according to the Vedas (Indian scriptures) produces energy.

Studies have shown the beneficial effects of yoga not only in stress and lifestyle-related diseases but also in the management of pain-related conditions. In two different studies, yoga therapy for three months and the use of transcendental meditation demonstrated a significant reduction in frequency and severity of pain in migraine patients.

Find a yoga teacher who uses a more traditional approach, rather than one that resembles aerobics that often features in modern yoga studios. It is not about fitness, flexibility and strength, but about putting yourself into positions that activate your energetic system in a particular manner.

Breathing

Breathing is another way to detoxify our bodies. We flush out carbon dioxide and bring in fresh oxygen, which bathes our tissues. Oxygen is alkaline and anti-inflammatory, and eliminates viruses. When we are stressed or traumatised, we often display dysregulated breathing. Focusing on our breath can bring us into the present moment and allow a pathway to regulation.

Hyperbaric chambers are useful for stimulating healing processes as they increase oxygenated blood flow to our organs, improving wound healing and healing infections, especially in oxygen-starved tissue. Hyperbaric oxygen therapy dissolves oxygen directly into the blood plasma, enabling higher levels of oxygen to reach areas where circulation is diminished or obstructed as a consequence of disease or injury. This non-invasive and painless treatment can reduce swelling in acute injuries, stimulate the growth of new blood vessels in tissues that have inadequate blood circulation, and boost the immune system in fighting certain types of infections. We can't always be living in hyperbaric chambers to stimulate our oxygen flow in our body, so best we learn how to breathe. Let's check in on your breathing on this quick test.

 Task

Place your left hand over your navel and your right hand over your chest.

Breathe normally (however you usually breathe, without thinking about it).

Which hand(s) is moving? Left, right, or both? If the hand over your chest is moving, you probably have a shallow breath.

That is, you're drawing insufficient oxygen when you breathe. This leads to fatigue and increases the chances of feeling anxiety.

If the hand over your navel is moving, you're probably breathing properly. This is called diaphragmatic breathing.

Breath is the first act of life and when we breathe well, we wash our bodies and organs with oxygen. When there is stress or anxiety, our breath may become restricted. Breath is the main source of prana – the vital life force for our energy system to operate. Breathing affects all of our bodily systems, feelings and moods in profound ways. In an age where most humans are in a constant state of anxiety, with overactivation of the sympathetic nervous system, proper breathing is a healthy way to reduce anxiety, restlessness and stress. By activating the parasympathetic nervous system, proper breathing promotes inner calm and physical relaxation.

The brain uses up to three times more oxygen than our muscles. The amount of oxygen in our bloodstream improves with proper breathing, increasing the amount of oxygen available to the brain.

This enhances brain function, translating to increased physical energy, mental clarity and productivity. By learning to direct your attention to your breath, you can condition yourself to shift out of stressful, depressed and aggressive mental states and enter relaxed, calm and resourceful states. The immediate advantages are clear: you become better equipped at handling challenging circumstances, managing conflict and retaining focus while working. Long-term advantages of good breathing include increased longevity and a better quality of life since it enhances your body's response to stress. Here are a few suggestions for better breathing:

- Breathe deeply with your belly or diaphragm instead of your chest (chest breathing can promote anxiety and emotional imbalance; belly breathing promotes relaxation). Visualise filling your whole body up with oxygen.
- Inhale through the nose as it purifies the air.
- Breathe steadily and rhythmically, lengthening your inhalations and exhalations without strain and matching the length of your exhalations to the length of your inhalations.
- Breathe slowly and quietly.
- Check in with your breath throughout the day. As we get stressed, our breathing tends to get shallower.
- Use breathing techniques when you are stressed.

Art of Living or Inner Engineering are accessible places to begin. These are systems of yogic methods known as kriya and incorporate pranayama. Art of Living uses something called Surdarshan Kriya, which is a powerful rhythmic breathing technique that incorporates specific natural rhythms of the breath, harmonising the body, mind and emotions. The technique is believed to eliminate stress, fatigue and negative emotions, such as anger, frustration and depression, leaving the mind calm and focused and the body energised and relaxed. It is a daily practice. People who practise it report better immunity, increased stamina and sustained high energy levels. I highly recommend doing one of these courses – they have a profound effect on body and mind.

Here are some breathing techniques to help you manage during times of stress:

1. The huff cough
   - Place yourself in a comfortable seated position. Inhale through your mouth, slightly more deeply than you would when taking a normal breath.
   - Activate your stomach muscles to blow the air out in three even breaths while making the sound 'ha, ha, ha'. Imagine you're blowing onto a mirror to cause it to steam up.

2. Alternate nostril breathing
   This is typically taught in yoga classes as a pranayama. It may be useful to get a yoga practitioner to guide you here. To practice alternate nostril breathing:
   - Sit in a comfortable position with your legs crossed.
   - Place your left hand on your left knee.
   - Lift your right hand up to your nose.
   - Exhale completely and then use your right thumb to close your right nostril.
   - Inhale through your left nostril for a count of four, then close the left nostril with your pinkie and ring fingers.
   - Open the right nostril and exhale through this side, for a count of six.

- Inhale through the right nostril for a count of four, and then close this nostril.
- Open the left nostril and exhale through this side for a count of six.
- This is one cycle.
- Continue for up to five minutes.
- Always complete the practice by finishing with an exhalation on the left side.

3. Pursed-lip breathing

This technique stimulates the parasympathetic nervous system. Use this technique when you are feeling anxious or overwhelmed:

- Keeping your mouth closed, take a deep breath in through your nose, counting to four. The breath doesn't have to be deep. A typical inhalation will do.
- Put your lips together as if you're starting to whistle or blow out candles on a birthday cake. This is known as pursing your lips.
- Keeping your lips pursed, slowly breathe out by counting to six. Don't try to force the air out; just breathe out slowly through your mouth.

4. 4–6–8 breathing

This is a specific pattern that involves holding the breath for a period to allow your body to replenish its oxygen. It forces the mind and body to focus on regulating the breath, rather than on replaying your worries. Find a place to sit or lie down comfortably. If you're using the technique to fall asleep, lying down is best. Rest the tip of your tongue against the roof of your mouth, right behind your top front teeth. Keep your tongue in place throughout the practice.

Do the following steps in the cycle of one breath:

- Exhale completely through your mouth.
- Close your lips, inhaling silently through your nose for the count of four.
- Then, for six seconds, hold your breath.
- Exhale for the count of eight.
- When you inhale again, you initiate a new cycle of breath. Practise this pattern for four full breaths.

The held breath is the most critical part of this practice. Do this for four breaths only when you're first starting out, then gradually work your way up to eight breaths.

Meditation

Meditation is a practice in which you use a technique – such as mindfulness, or focusing the mind on a particular object, thought or activity – to train attention and awareness, and achieve a mentally clear and emotionally calm and stable state. The aim is to harness a tranquil mind. According to Buddhist principles, the 'monkey mind' is a term that refers to being unsettled, restless or confused. It is also the part of your brain that becomes easily distracted, so if you want to get anything done in life, your challenge will be to shut down the monkey mind. Restless thoughts lead to restless, chaotic action, as what is internal manifests externally. Meditation can be a brave introspective process that can also aid the psychotherapeutic journey. If you struggle to sit still, using qigong, yoga or kriya as a meditation may accommodate your more kinaesthetic nature.

For chronic conditions, I recommend a body scan meditation. There are many guided ones on YouTube that you can use until you are able to guide yourself through it. This can be an ideal way of learning to tune into the body more effectively and feel what it needs from you. It can also be a way to identify symptoms and sit with them in a way that does not elicit anxiety. At the start of my journey, each of my symptoms would elicit a cascade of fear. I have now made friends with my symptoms as useful messengers.

A sound journey can be a form of meditation, and I recommend finding practitioners who do these. Practitioners can work with voice, quartz crystals, singing bowls, gongs, flutes, drums, and a variety of other instruments to create a soundscape for your journey. They can elicit things that need to be worked through or put you into a deeply restful state. Sound is a frequency and has the power to shift and heal your energetic frequency. This is why shamans use this tool.

Temperature-based healing

Steam baths, saunas, hot yoga and cold-water immersion can all benefit the detoxification pathways and stimulate the immune system. Infrared sauna is popular in the treatment of autoimmune conditions as it can help improve circulation, reduce inflammation, enhance the detoxification process, and more. Cold-water bathing stimulates our immune system, causing a form of evolutionary stress that makes the immune system work harder and more efficiently to protect us not only from the effects of cooling in cold weather but also from infection by bacteria and viruses. The immune system becomes more robust and effective, and quicker to respond. So, brief, daily cold baths may boost immune function. For more about this, read up about the Wim Hof Method.

Be gentle with yourself not to put additional strain on the body and remember to listen to your body if these do not feel good. In the case of the hot remedies, don't forget to hydrate!

PART 4

❧

Endings

ILLNESS COMES INTO your life to reshape you, if you allow it. It gives you another lease on life. It increases the value of your own life and of the lives of others, if you let it. It introduces an openness to re-evaluation and flexibility in your life as a permanent feature. If you can liberate yourself once, you will never get stuck again. The biggest stress in life is not being who you truly are, and illness comes to bring you to your authentic self.

Your job is to be open to illness and support your body with any of the methods provided here that resonate with you. Stick to a diet that works for your body – more than half of the difficulties with autoimmune conditions can be resolved with the correct nutrition. Hippocrates states that your food should be your medicine – these words are believed to have come from Ayurveda. Detoxify, clean and strengthen your body, increase nutrient delivery, and harmonise your immune system.

Animals have an instinctive nature in that they know what they need to do – when they need to rest, sleep, eat and be in community. All autoimmune diseases involve disconnection from the body, which is a result of trauma. Work through and regulate yourself off your stress and trauma. Reconnecting to your body will allow you to better meet your physical needs.

Remember our connection to plants. Start an intuitive and symbiotic relationship with herbs. Much of what I have discussed in this book speaks about our relationship to natural plant-based medicine – Ayurveda, TCM, diet and ayahuasca. Learn to relate to others in a way that does not take away from you. Create a healing protocol for yourself, which you can start to formulate from the brief notes you have made in this book. Keep motivated, disciplined and hopeful, but don't be hard on yourself – your body will feel it.

Simplify your life, adapt and flow with change. Let go of the need to control, turn complaints into gratitude, and recognise that you are already perfect and that there is no need to change or improve yourself. Just love who you have always been.

This book contains a lot of information – a lot to integrate right now, perhaps. You may already have realised most of this intuitively; maybe you are already far along this path. Wherever you are in this process, do what you can and do what feels best. It is not about perfection: perhaps striving for perfection is one of those qualities that led you here to begin with.

Stick with nature and live as naturally as possible, like our ancestors used to. This, in essence, is what we need to heal; these illnesses are our soul craving to come back to a natural life and connection with all living beings.

References and recommended reading

Allen, B. G., Bhatia, S. K., Anderson, C. M., Eichenberger-Gilmore, J. M., Sibenaller, Z.A., Mapuskar, K. A., Schoenfeld, J. D., Buatti, J. M., Spitz, D. R., & Fath, M. A. (2014). Ketogenic diets as an adjuvant cancer therapy: History and potential mechanism. *Redox Biology*, 2, 963–970. https://doi.org/10.1016/j.redox.2014.08.002

Barbaro, B., Toietta, G., Maggio, R., Arciello, M., Tarocchi, M., Galli, A., & Balsano, C. (2014). Effects of the olive-derived polyphenol oleuropein on human health. *International Journal of Molecular Sciences*, 15(10), 18508–18524. https://doi.org/10.3390/ijms151018508

BBC. (2022). Research finds nature sounds 'benefit mental health'. https://www.bbc.com/news/uk-england-devon-60840759

Berceli, D., & Scaer, R. (2015). *Shake It Off Naturally: Reduce Stress, Anxiety, and Tension with [TRE]*. Create Space Independent Publishing.

Bjørklund, G., Dadar, M., Pen, J. J., Chirumbolo, S., & Aaseth, J. (2019). Chronic fatigue syndrome (CFS): Suggestions for a nutritional treatment in the therapeutic approach. *Biomedicine & Pharmacotherapy*, 109, 1000–1007. https://doi.org/10.1016/j.biopha.2018.10.076

Blum, W. E. H., Zechmeister-Boltenstern, S., & Keiblinger, K. M. (2019). Does Soil Contribute to the Human Gut Microbiome? *Microorganisms*, 7(9), 287. https://doi.org/10.3390/microorganisms7090287

Bohacek, J., & Mansuy, I. M. (2013). Epigenetic inheritance of disease and disease risk. *Neuropsychopharmacology: Official publication of the American College of Neuropsychopharmacology*, 38(1), 220–236. https://doi.org/10.1038/npp.2012.110

Boulis, M., Boulis, M., & Clauw, D. (2021). Magnesium and Fibromyalgia: A Literature Review. *Journal of Primary Care & Community Health*, 12, 21501327211038433. https://doi.org/10.1177/21501327211038433

Brand, M. D., Orr, A. L., Perevoshchikova, I. V., & Quinlan, C. L. (2013). The role of mitochondrial function and cellular bioenergetics in ageing and disease. *The British Journal of Dermatology*, 169 Suppl 2(0 2), 1–8. https://doi.org/10.1111/bjd.12208

Brooks, H. L., Rushton, K., Lovell, K., Bee, P., Walker, L., Grant, L., & Rogers, A. (2018). *The power of support from companion animals for people living with mental health problems: A systematic review and narrative synthesis of the evidence*. BMC Psychiatry, 18(1), 31. https://doi.org/10.1186/s12888-018-1613-2

Buxton, R. T., Pearson, A. L., Allou, C., Fristrup, K., & Wittemyer, G. (2021). A synthesis of health benefits of natural sounds and their distribution in national parks. *Proceedings of the National Academy of Sciences of the United States of America*, 118(14), e2013097118. https://doi.org/10.1073/pnas.2013097118

Cannon, W. (1957). 'Voodoo' death. *Psychosomatic Medicine*, 19, 182–190.

Carbonaro, T. M., & Gatch, M. B. (2016). Neuropharmacology of N,N-dimethyltryptamine. *Brain Research Bulletin*, 126(Pt 1), 74–88. https://doi.org/10.1016/j.brainresbull.2016.04.016

Ceci, L. (2022). Average unlocks per day among smartphone users in the United States as of August 2018, by generation. https://www.statista.com/statistics/1050339/average-unlocks-per-day-us-smartphone-users/

Ceccarelli, F., Agmon-Levin, N., & Perricone, C. (2016). Genetic Factors of Autoimmune Diseases. *Journal of Immunology Research*, 2016, 3476023. https://doi.org/10.1155/2016/3476023

Chen, L., Deng, H., Cui, H., Fang, J., Zuo, Z., Deng, J., Li, Y., Wang, X., & Zhao, L. (2017).

Inflammatory responses and inflammation-associated diseases in organs. Oncotarget, 9(6), 7204–7218. https://doi.org/10.18632/oncotarget.23208

Chevalier, G., Sinatra, S. T., Oschman, J. L., Sokal, K., & Sokal, P. (2012). Earthing: Health implications of reconnecting the human body to the Earth's surface electrons. *Journal of Environmental and Public Health*, 2012, 291541. https://doi.org/10.1155/2012/291541

Chong, C. S., Tsunaka, M., Tsang, H. W., Chan, E. P., & Cheung, W. M. (2011). Effects of yoga on stress management in healthy adults: A systematic review. *Alternative Therapies in Health and Medicine*, 17(1), 32–38.

Crosby, L., Davis, B., Joshi, S., Jardine, M., Paul, J., Neola, M., & Barnard, N. D. (2021). Ketogenic Diets and Chronic Disease: Weighing the Benefits Against the Risks. *Frontiers in Nutrition*, 8, 702802. https://doi.org/10.3389/fnut.2021.702802

Coviello, A. W. (2015). *The Medical Medium*. Hay House.

Cox, I. M., Campbell, M. J., & Dowson, D. (1991). Red blood cell magnesium and chronic fatigue syndrome. *The Lancet*, 337(8744), 757–760. https://doi.org/10.1016/0140-6736(91)91371-z

Cunningham, S. (2018). The hidden stress of cell phones. UCHealth. https://www.uchealth.org/today/the-hidden-stress-of-cell-phones/

Damasio, A. (1999). *The Feeling of What Happens: Body and emotion in the making of consciousness*. New York: Harcourt, Brace.

D'Andrea Meira, I., Romão, T. T., Pires do Prado, H. J., Krüger, L. T., Pires, M. E. P., & Da Conceição, P. O. (2019). Ketogenic Diet and Epilepsy: What We Know So Far. *Frontiers in Neuroscience*, 13, 5. https://doi.org/10.3389/fnins.2019.00005

DeQuattro, K., Trupin, L., Li, J., Katz, P. P., Murphy, L. B., Yelin, E. H., Rush, S., Lanata, C., Criswell, L. A., Dall'Era, M., & Yazdany, J. (2020). Relationships Between Adverse Childhood Experiences and Health Status in Systemic Lupus Erythematosus. *Arthritis Care & Research*, 72(4), 525–533. https://doi.org/10.1002/acr.23878

Denham-Jones, L., Gaskell, L., Spence, N., & Pigott, T. (2022). A systematic review of the effectiveness of yoga on pain, physical function, and quality of life in older adults with chronic musculoskeletal conditions. *Musculoskeletal Care*, 20(1), 47–73. https://doi.org/10.1002/msc.1576

Dienes, K. A., Hammen, C., Henry, R. M., Cohen, A. N., & Daley, S. E. (2006). The stress sensitization hypothesis: Understanding the course of bipolar disorder. *Journal of Affective Disorders*, 95(1–3), 43–49. https://doi.org/10.1016/j.jad.2006.04.009

Dube, S. R., Fairweather, D., Pearson, W. S., Felitti, V. J., Anda, R. F., & Croft, J. B. (2009). Cumulative childhood stress and autoimmune diseases in adults. *Psychosomatic Medicine*, 71(2), 243–250. https://doi.org/10.1097/PSY.0b013e3181907888

Engel, G.I. (1971). Sudden and rapid death during psychological stress: Folklore or wisdom? *Annals of Internal Medicine*, 74, 771–782.

Felitti, V., & Anda, R. (2010). The relationship of adverse childhood experiences to adult medical disease, psychiatric disorders and sexual behavior: Implications for healthcare. In R. Lanius, E. Vermetten, & C. Pain (Eds.). *The Impact of Early Life Trauma on Health and Disease: The hidden epidemic* (pp. 77–87). Cambridge University Press. doi:10.1017/CBO9780511777042.010

Gilden, D. H. (2005). Infectious causes of multiple sclerosis. *The Lancet*. Neurology, 4(3), 195–202. https://doi.org/10.1016/S1474-4422(05)01017-3

Gold, J. E., Okyay, R. A., Licht, W. E., & Hurley, D. J. (2021). Investigation of long COVID prevalence and its relationship to Epstein-Barr virus reactivation. *Pathogens*, 10(6). doi:

10.3390/pathogens10060763

Harpaz, I., Abutbul, S., Nemirovsky, A., Gal, R., Cohen, H., & Monsonego, A. (2013). Chronic exposure to stress predisposes to higher autoimmune susceptibility in C57BL/6 mice: Glucocorticoids as a double-edged sword. *European Journal of Immunology*, 43(3), 758–769. https://doi.org/10.1002/eji.201242613

Haddad, H. W., Mallepalli, N. R., Scheinuk, J. E., Bhargava, P., Cornett, E. M., Urits, I., & Kaye, A. D. (2021). The Role of Nutrient Supplementation in the Management of Chronic Pain in Fibromyalgia: A Narrative Review. *Pain and Therapy*, 10(2), 827–848. https://doi.org/10.1007/s40122-021-00266-9

Hammen, C., Henry, R., & Daley, S. E. (2000). Depression and sensitization to stressors among young women as a function of childhood adversity. *Journal of Consulting and Clinical Psychology*, 68(5), 782–787.

Hay, L. (1999). *You Can Heal Your Life*. Carlsbad, CA: Hay House.

Hernandez-Reif, M., Field, T., Ironson, G., Beutler, J., Vera, Y., Hurley, J., Fletcher, M. A., Schanberg, S., Kuhn, C., & Fraser, M. (2005). Natural killer cells and lymphocytes increase in women with breast cancer following massage therapy. *The International Journal of Neuroscience*, 115(4), 495–510. https://doi.org/10.1080/00207450590523080

Hewagama, A., & Richardson, B. (2009). The genetics and epigenetics of autoimmune diseases. *Journal of Autoimmunity*, 33(1), 3–11. https://doi.org/10.1016/j.jaut.2009.03.007

Judith, A. (2004). *Eastern Body, Western Mind: Psychology and the chakra system as a path to the self*. Berkeley, CA: Celestial Arts.

Joel, N. G. (2020). It Takes Guts: Psychedelic Treatment Approaches to Autoimmune Disorders. *Psychedelic Science Review*. https://psychedelicreview.com/it-takes-guts-psychedelic-treatment-approaches-to-autoimmune-disorders/

Kaplan, T. B., Berkowitz, A. L., & Samuels, M. A. (2015). Cardiovascular Dysfunction in Multiple Sclerosis. *The Neurologist*, 20(6), 108–114. https://doi.org/10.1097/NRL.0000000000000064

Kim, S. K., & Bae, H. (2010). Acupuncture and immune modulation. *Autonomic Neuroscience: Basic & Clinical*, 157(1–2), 38–41. https://doi.org/10.1016/j.autneu.2010.03.010

King University. (2017). Cell Phone Addiction: The Statistics of Gadget Dependency. https://online.king.edu/news/cell-phone-addiction/

Klement, R. J. (2019). The emerging role of ketogenic diets in cancer treatment. *Current Opinion in Clinical Nutrition and Metabolic Care*, 22(2), 129–134. https://doi.org/10.1097/MCO.0000000000000540

Kosinski, C., & Jornayvaz, F. R. (2017). Effects of Ketogenic Diets on Cardiovascular Risk Factors: Evidence from Animal and Human Studies. *Nutrients*, 9(5), 517. https://doi.org/10.3390/nu9050517

Lacal, I., & Ventura, R. (2018). Epigenetic Inheritance: Concepts, Mechanisms and Perspectives. *Frontiers in Molecular Neuroscience*, 11, 292. https://doi.org/10.3389/fnmol.2018.00292

Levine, P. (1997). *Waking the Tiger: Healing trauma*. Berkeley, CA: North Atlantic Books.

Levine, P. A. (2010). *In an Unspoken Voice: How the body releases trauma and restores goodness*. Berkeley, CA: North Atlantic Books.

Li, N., Guo, Y., Gong, Y., Zhang, Y., Fan, W., Yao, K., Chen, Z., Dou, B., Lin, X., Chen, B., Chen, Z., Xu, Z., & Lyu, Z. (2021). The Anti-Inflammatory Actions and Mechanisms of Acupuncture from Acupoint to Target Organs via Neuro-Immune Regulation. *Journal of Inflammation Research*, 4, 7191–7224. https://doi.org/10.2147/JIR.S341581

Li, Q., Morimoto, K., Nakadai, A., Inagaki, H., Katsumata, M., Shimizu, T., Hirata, Y., Hirata, K., Suzuki, H., Miyazaki, Y., Kagawa, T., Koyama, Y., Ohira, T., Takayama, N., Krensky, A. M., & Kawada, T. (2007). Forest bathing enhances human natural killer activity and expression of anti-cancer proteins. *International Journal of Immunopathology and Pharmacology*, 20(2 Suppl 2), 3–8. https://doi.org/10.1177/03946320070200S202

Li, Q. Q., Shi, G. X., Xu, Q., Wang, J., Liu, C. Z., & Wang, L. P. (2013). Acupuncture effect and central autonomic regulation. *Evidence-based Complementary and Alternative Medicine: eCAM*, 2013, 267959. https://doi.org/10.1155/2013/267959

Li, A. W., & Goldsmith, C. A. (2012). The effects of yoga on anxiety and stress. *Alternative Medicine Review: A Journal of Clinical Therapeutic*, 17(1), 21–35.

Li, S., Yu, Y., Yue, Y., Zhang, Z., & Su, K. (2013). Microbial Infection and Rheumatoid Arthritis. *Journal of Clinical & Cellular Immunology*, 4(6), 174. https://doi.org/10.4172/2155-9899.1000174

Liu, M., Yu, S., Wang, J., Qiao, J., Liu, Y., Wang, S., & Zhao, Y. (2020). Ginseng protein protects against mitochondrial dysfunction and neurodegeneration by inducing mitochondrial unfolded protein response in Drosophila melanogaster PINK1 model of Parkinson's disease. *Journal of Ethnopharmacology*, 247, 112213. https://doi.org/10.1016/j.jep.2019.112213

Macarenco, M. M., Opariuc-Dan, C., & Nedelcea, C. (2021). Childhood trauma, dissociation, alexithymia, and anger in people with autoimmune diseases: A mediation model. *Child Abuse & Neglect*, 122, 105322. https://doi.org/10.1016/j.chiabu.2021.105322

Maia, L. O., Daldegan-Bueno, D., & Tófoli, L. F. (2021). The ritual use of ayahuasca during treatment of severe physical illnesses: A qualitative study. *Journal of Psychoactive Drugs*, 53(3), 272–282. https://doi.org/10.1080/02791072.2020.1854399

Manoharan, S., & Ying, L. Y. (2023). Epstein Barr Virus Reactivation during COVID-19 Hospitalization Significantly Increased Mortality/Death in SARS-CoV-2(+)/EBV(+) than SARS-CoV-2(+)/EBV(-) Patients: A Comparative Meta-Analysis. *International Journal of Clinical Practice*, 2023, 1068000. https://doi.org/10.1155/2023/1068000

Marrodan, M., Alessandro, L., Farez, M. F., & Correale, J. (2019). The role of infections in multiple sclerosis. *Multiple Sclerosis*, 25(7), 891–901. https://doi.org/10.1177/1352458518823940

Maté, G. (2022). Authenticity Can Heal Trauma. https://www.madinamerica.com/2022/12/authenticity-can-heal-trauma-dr-gabor-mate-md/

Maté, G., & Maté, D. (2022). *The Myth of Normal*. USA: Penguin Random House

Maté, G. (2003). *When the Body Says No: The cost of hidden stress*. Carlton, Vic: Scribe Publications.

Mavropoulos, J. C., Yancy, W. S., Hepburn, J., & Westman, E. C. (2005). The effects of a low-carbohydrate, ketogenic diet on the polycystic ovary syndrome: A pilot study. *Nutrition & Metabolism*, 2, 35. https://doi.org/10.1186/1743-7075-2-35

Memme, J. M., Erlich, A. T., Phukan, G., & Hood, D. A. (2021). Exercise and mitochondrial health. *The Journal of Physiology*, 599(3), 803–817. https://doi.org/10.1113/JP278853

Milaneschi, Y., Kappelmann, N., Ye, Z. et al. Association of inflammation with depression and anxiety: Evidence for symptom-specificity and potential causality from UK Biobank and NESDA cohorts. *Molecular Psychiatry*, 26, 7393–7402 (2021). https://doi.org/10.1038/s41380-021-01188-w

Mincu, R. I., Magda, L. S., Florescu, M., Velcea, A., Mihaila, S., Mihalcea, D., Popescu, B. O., Chiru, A., Tiu, C., Cinteza, M., & Vinereanu, D. (2015). Cardiovascular Dysfunction in Multiple Sclerosis. *Maedica*, 10(4), 364–370.

Morhenn, V., Beavin, L. E., & Zak, P. J. (2012). Massage increases oxytocin and reduces adrenocorticotropin hormone in humans. *Alternative Therapies in Health and Medicine*, 18(6), 11–18.

Myss, C. (1996). *Anatomy of the Spirit: The seven stages of power and healing*. Harmony.

Nieman, D. C., & Wentz, L. M. (2019). The compelling link between physical activity and the body's defense system. *Journal of Sport and Health Science*, 8(3), 201–217. https://doi. org/10.1016/j.jshs.2018.09.009

Ogden, P., Minton, K., & Pain, C. (2006). *Trauma and the Body: A sensorimotor approach to psychotherapy*. W. W. Norton & Company.

Ogle, C. M., Rubin, D. C., & Siegler, I. C. (2013). The impact of the developmental timing of trauma exposure on PTSD symptoms and psychosocial functioning among older adults. *Developmental Psychology*, 49(11), 2191–2200. https://doi.org/10.1037/a0031985

Pacini, F., Vorontsova, T., Molinaro, E., Shavrova, E., Agate, L., Kuchinskaya, E., Elisei, R., Demidchik, E. P., & Pinchera, A. (1999). Thyroid consequences of the Chernobyl nuclear accident. *Acta Paediatrica*, Supplement, 88(433), 23–27. https://doi.org/10.1111/j.1651-2227.1999.tb14399.x

Peluso, M. J., Deveau, T. M., Munter, S. E., Ryder, D., Buck, A., Beck-Engeser, G., Chan, F., Lu, S., Goldberg, S. A., Hoh, R., Tai, V., Torres, L., Iyer, N. S., Deswal, M., Ngo, L. H., Buitrago, M., Rodriguez, A., Chen, J. Y., Yee, B. C., Chenna, A., … Henrich, T. J. (2022). Impact of Pre-Existing Chronic Viral Infection and Reactivation on the Development of Long COVID. *medRxiv: The Preprint Server for Health Sciences*, 2022.06.21.22276660. https://doi.org/10.1101/2022.06.21.22276660

Pavlov, I. (1966). *Essential Works of Pavlov* (M. Kaplan, Ed.). New York, NY: Bantam.

Porges, S. W. (2011). *The Polyvagal Theory: Neurophysiological foundations of emotions, attachment, communication, self-regulation*. New York, NY: Norton.

Pucadyil, T. J., Chipuk, J. E., Liu, Y., O'Neill, L., & Chen, Q. (2023). The multifaceted roles of mitochondria. *Molecular Cell*, 83(6), 819–823. https://doi.org/10.1016/j.molcel.2023.02.030

Rapaport, M. H., Schettler, P., & Bresee, C. (2012). A preliminary study of the effects of repeated massage on hypothalamic-pituitary-adrenal and immune function in healthy individuals: A study of mechanisms of action and dosage. *Journal of Alternative and Complementary Medicine*, 18(8), 789–797. https://doi.org/10.1089/acm.2011.0071

Ravan, J. R., Chatterjee, S., Singh, P., Maikap, D., & Padhan, P. (2021). Autoimmune Rheumatic Diseases Masquerading as Psychiatric Disorders: A Case Series. *Mediterranean Journal of Rheumatology*, 32(2), 164–167. https://doi.org/10.31138/mjr.32.2.164

Richter, C. (1957). On the phenomenon of sudden death in animals and man. *Psychosomatic Medicine*, 19, 191–198.

Rodríguez, Y., Rojas, M., Beltrán, S., Polo, F., Camacho-Domínguez, L., Morales, S. D., Gershwin, M. E., & Anaya, J. M. (2022). Autoimmune and autoinflammatory conditions after COVID-19 vaccination. New case reports and updated literature review. *Journal of autoimmunity*, 132, 102898. https://doi.org/10.1016/j.jaut.2022.102898

Romero-Márquez, J. M., Forbes-Hernández, T. Y., Navarro-Hortal, M. D., Quirantes-Piné, R., Grosso, G., Giampieri, F., Lipari, V., Sánchez-González, C., Battino, M., & Quiles, J. L. (2023). Molecular Mechanisms of the Protective Effects of Olive Leaf Polyphenols against Alzheimer's Disease. *International Journal of Molecular Sciences*, 24(5), 4353. https://doi. org/10.3390/ijms24054353

Rothschild, B. (2000). *The Body Remembers: The psychophysiology of trauma and trauma treatment*. W. W. Norton & Company.

Rothschild, B. (2010). *8 Keys to Safe Trauma Recovery: Take-charge strategies to empower your healing.* New York, NY: Norton.

Rusek, M., Pluta, R., Ułamek-Kozioł, M., & Czuczwar, S. J. (2019). Ketogenic Diet in Alzheimer's Disease. *International Journal of Molecular Sciences*, 20(16), 3892. https://doi.org/10.3390/ijms20163892

Saul, L. (1966). Sudden death at impasse. *Psychological Forum*, 1, 88–89.

Scaer, R. (2005). *The Trauma Spectrum: Hidden wounds and human resiliency.* New York, NY: Norton.

Scaer, R. C. (2007). *The Body Bears the Burden: Trauma, dissociation and disease* (2nd ed.). New York, NY: Routledge, Taylor & Francis Group.

Schore, A. N. (1994). *Affect Regulation and the Origin of the Self: The neurobiology of emotional development.* Hillsdale, NJ: Lawrence Erlbaum.

Selye, H. (1958). The Stress of Life. New York, NY: McGraw-Hill.

Schmid, J., Jungaberle, H., & Verres, R. (2010). Subjective Theories About (Self-) Treatment with Ayahuasca. *Anthropology of Consciousness*, 21, 188–204. 10.1111/j.1556-3537.2010.01028.x.

Schmid, J. T. (2014). Healing with Ayahuasca: Notes on Therapeutic Rituals and Effects in European Patients Treating Their Diseases. In B. C. Labate & C. Cavnar (Eds). *The Therapeutic Use of Ayahuasca.* Springer, Berlin, Heidelberg. https://doi.org/10.1007/978-3-642-40426-9_5

Shapiro, D. (2012). *The Body Speaks Your Mind.* Brown Book Group.

Siegel, D. J. (2006). An Interpersonal Neurobiology Approach to Psychotherapy: Awareness, Mirror Neurons, and Neural Plasticity in the Development of Well-Being. *Psychiatric Annals*, 36. 10.3928/00485713-20060401-06.

Siegel, D. J. (2007). *The Mindful Brain: Reflection and attunement in the cultivation of well-being.* New York, NY: Norton.

Siegel, D. J. (2020). *The Developing Mind: How relationships and the brain interact to shape who we are* (3rd ed.). The Guilford Press.

Sloka, S., Silva, C., Pryse-Phillips, W., Patten, S., Metz, L., & Yong, V. (2011). A Quantitative Analysis of Suspected Environmental Causes of MS. *Canadian Journal of Neurological Sciences*, 38(1), 98–105. doi:10.1017/S0317167100011124

Skinner, M. K. (2014). A new kind of inheritance. *Scientific American*, 311(2), 44–51. https://doi.org/10.1038/scientificamerican0814-44

Song, H., Fang, F., Tomasson, G., Arnberg, F. K., Mataix-Cols, D., Fernández de la Cruz, L., Almqvist, C., Fall, K., & Valdimarsdóttir, U. A. (2018). Association of Stress-Related Disorders With Subsequent Autoimmune Disease. JAMA, 319(23), 2388–2400. https://doi.org/10.1001/jama.2018.7028

Stocker, R. K., Reber Aubry, E., Bally, L., Nuoffer, J. M., & Stanga, Z. (2019). Ketogene Diät: evidenzbasierte therapeutische Anwendung bei endokrinologischen Erkrankungen [Ketogenic Diet and its Evidence-Based Therapeutic Implementation in Endocrine Diseases]. *Praxis*, 108(8), 541–553. https://doi.org/10.1024/1661-8157/a003246

Stojanovich, L. (2010). Stress and autoimmunity. *Autoimmunity Reviews*, 9(5), A271–A276. https://doi.org/10.1016/j.autrev.2009.11.014

Stojanovich, L., & Marisavljevich, D. (2008). Stress as a trigger of autoimmune disease. *Autoimmunity Reviews*, 7(3), 209–213. https://doi.org/10.1016/j.autrev.2007.11.007

Thompson, C., & Szabo, A. (2020). Psychedelics as a novel approach to treating autoimmune conditions. *Immunology Letters*, 228, 45–54. https://doi.org/10.1016/j.imlet.2020.10.001

Tripathi, M. N., Kumari, S., & Ganpat, T. S. (2018). Psychophysiological effects of yoga on stress in college students. *Journal of Education and Health Promotion*, 7, 43. https://doi.org/10.4103/jehp.jehp_74_17

Tolle, E. (2016). *The Power of Now: A guide to spiritual enlightenment.* Yellow Kite.

Van der Kolk, B. A., & Pratt, S. (2014). *The Body Keeps the Score: Brain, mind, and body in the healing of trauma.* New York, NY: Gildan Media.

Wens, I., Dalgas, U., Stenager, E., & Eijnde, B. O. (2013). Risk factors related to cardiovascular diseases and the metabolic syndrome in multiple sclerosis: A systematic review. *Multiple Sclerosis,* 19(12), 1556–1564. https://doi.org/10.1177/1352458513504252

Wentz, I. (2017). *Hashimoto's Protocol: A 90-day plan for reversing thyroid symptoms and getting your life back.* New York, NY: HarperCollins.

White, G. E., West, S. L., Caterini, J. E., Di Battista, A. P., Rhind, S. G., & Wells, G. D. (2020). Massage Therapy Modulates Inflammatory Mediators Following Sprint Exercise in Healthy Male Athletes. *Journal of Functional Morphology and Kinesiology,* 5(1), 9. https://doi.org/10.3390/jfmk5010009

Wren, A. A., Wright, M. A., Carson, J. W., & Keefe, F. J. (2011). Yoga for persistent pain: New findings and directions for an ancient practice. *Pain,* 152(3), 477–480. https://doi.org/10.1016/j.pain.2010.11.017

Yahyapour, R., Amini, P., Rezapour, S., Cheki, M., Rezaeyan, A., Farhood, B., Shabeeb, D., Musa, A. E., Fallah, H., & Najafi, M. (2018). Radiation-induced inflammation and autoimmune diseases. *Military Medical Research,* 5(1), 9. https://doi.org/10.1186/s40779-018-0156-7